HEARING BEETHOVEN

Hearing Beethoven

A STORY OF MUSICAL LOSS
AND DISCOVERY

Robin Wallace

THE UNIVERSITY OF CHICAGO PRESS

CHICAGO AND LONDON

The University of Chicago Press, Chicago 60637

The University of Chicago Press, Ltd., London

© 2018 by The University of Chicago

Published 2018

Printed in the United States of America

27 26 25 24 23 22 21 20 19 18   1 2 3 4 5

ISBN-13: 978-0-226-42975-5 (cloth)

ISBN-13: 978-0-226-42989-2 (e-book)

DOI: https://doi.org/10.7208/chicago/9780226429892.001.0001

Library of Congress Cataloging-in-Publication Data

Names: Wallace, Robin, author.

Title: Hearing Beethoven : a story of musical loss and discovery / Robin Wallace.

Description: Chicago ; London : The University of Chicago Press, 2018. | Includes bibliographical references and index.

Identifiers: LCCN 2017060714 | ISBN 9780226429755 (cloth : alk. paper) | ISBN 9780226429892 (e-book)

Subjects: LCSH: Beethoven, Ludwig van, 1770-1827—Health. | Deafness.

Classification: LCC ML410.B4 W27 2018 | DDC 780.92—dc23

LC record available at https://lccn.loc.gov/2017060714

♾ This paper meets the requirements of ANSI/NISO Z39.48-1992 (Permanence of Paper).

In loving memory of Barbara,
and to Meg, whose love speaks through these pages

Contents

Preface

The old man walks stiffly onto the stage, just three days short of his eighty-fifth birthday. He looks frail but formidable, and when the camera cuts to his face his features are the stuff of legend. With his right hand he sweeps the baton in a 360-degree arc of fierce efficiency, his left hand mimicking it with only his index finger to carve the air, his chin and chiseled nose bending into the gesture so his whole body gives the downbeat. There is no sound. As the famous opening notes of Beethoven's Fifth Symphony predictably follow, Arturo Toscanini barely moves. With a dismissive gesture of his left hand, he silences the orchestra so he can start it once more.

The most familiar beginning in music does not speak all of its secrets to those who can only hear.

In the pages that follow I will invite the reader into the creative world of Ludwig van Beethoven, the most famous deaf musician in history. The fact that Beethoven continued to compose music after he lost his hearing has been presented as an act of heroism or a miracle of ingenuity. These are powerful ideas, but by demystifying what Beethoven did we can make him more human and his music more understandable. His deafness was a devastating blow, as it would be for any musician. It did not stop him from writing music, because music also grows from sight and touch. It emerges from the body and from instruments that move and vibrate. It responds to cues that can be seen, and it includes gestures that appeal as much to the eye as to the ear. Beethoven knew all this, and as his hearing failed he became more, not less, attached to the physical and visual dimensions of his craft.

I am in a unique position to tell this story because I lived for eight and a half years with someone who was profoundly deaf: my late wife Barbara, who inhabits the pages of this book along with Beethoven. I watched her frustrations and her triumphs and learned from her about my own humanity. From her example, I became convinced that Beethoven's response to his deafness was a natural part of human experience, that he was not a freak of nature.

As a pianist, Beethoven worked throughout his life with the complex technological marvel of the piano, a box fronted by keys that could be pushed and released and filled with hammers that sprang up in response and then mysteriously retreated. As a composer, he struggled to make music permanent: to affix it to paper with pen and pencil so he could shape it according to his will. Fortunately he left behind extensive records of this creative work in the form of sketches and manuscripts, whose secrets scholars are only beginning to tease out nearly two centuries after his death.

Those secrets, though, are hidden in plain sight, and you don't need to have in-depth knowledge or know how to read music to see what Beethoven was doing. The very abundance of written material he left behind shows that composing was, for him, a visual process and a physical one. His proverbially messy handwriting means that his music was taking shape on paper, before his eyes and ours. He didn't simply remember the sound of music, "hear it in his head," and write it down. He worked it out in intricate detail in writing because this was the way it increasingly made sense to compose. He also continued to work at the piano long after his ears had stopped receiving much benefit. The keys were still responsive, the hammers still rose and receded, and the instrument still vibrated to his touch.

But Beethoven also played the piano with a resonator—a cupola of sheet metal—built to concentrate the sound. He pushed manufacturers to make their instruments louder. Clearly sound still had value to him, even in very small amounts. We should not assume that these were pathetic attempts to surmount his loss and recover "normal" hearing. Even with a cochlear implant, that marvel of modern technological ingenuity, Barbara could not hear normally; she simply learned to make the most of what auditory input she could get. Beethoven did the same. He accepted and worked with his compromised hearing while also taking advantage of every technological support available to him. As a result, he lived in one of the most fascinating creative environments in the history of any art. With all that has been written about Beethoven, that story has not yet been told.

A Road Trip to Texas

We drove that June day through western Alabama, Interstate 20 unfolding before us as late afternoon blurred into evening. *A Prairie Home Companion* played on the radio, and as I laughed at a series of atrocious "knock, knock" jokes ("Knock, knock." "Who's there?" "Dyslexic." "Dyslexic how?"), my wife Barbara grinned, her delight in my delight evident in the sympathy that played out on her features. We had been married fourteen abundant years, and a touch or a shared gesture could convey volumes. One cross-country move lay in our past, a two-year-old and a five-month-old packed into a Honda Civic with a terrified cat as we trekked from California to South Carolina in six-hour segments, each ending with a plunge into a motel swimming pool. Now, our eleven- and nine-year-olds left safely with my mother in Knoxville, we were preparing to search for a house in Waco, Texas, so I could begin my dream job: a senior faculty appointment in the School of Music at Baylor University. I was a musicologist specializing in the critical reception of the music of Ludwig van Beethoven. Barbara was a registered nurse. It was 2003, we were both forty-seven, and life had not been easy for either of us.

I had struggled through my twenties to overcome devastating depression—stemming from years of brutal bullying throughout my childhood—and complete my PhD in music history at Yale, only to have the job market in my field dry up and virtually disappear, leading to a decade of underemployment. My first marriage had dissolved under the pressure. In 1994, married to Barbara for over five years, I had finally found a tenure-track job at a small women's college I had never heard of, and with half my life behind me I made the journey to South Carolina to begin what I thought of as my real career.

As for Barbara, she had survived cancer—a malignant brain tumor diagnosed on her twenty-third birthday—and lost her first husband, a captain in the marines, in a senseless helicopter crash. When we met at thirty-two, we bonded instantly because our lives had been parallel struggles for survival and sanity. Our marriage was born of a determination to make sense of our mutually broken dreams.

Now, as our time in South Carolina drew to a close, one of those dreams had been achieved and another had been shattered irrevocably. By accepting the job at Baylor, I had reached the pinnacle of my professional career. Weeks later, Barbara suddenly became completely deaf. As she rode next to me now, trying to share my amusement, she heard nothing.

Barbara had been hard of hearing since long before I knew her. The tumor from her twenties had required immediate surgery followed by radiation therapy. Because of the location of the tumor—the right cerebellum—and complications from the surgery, the radiation had to be administered through her ears. That radiation saved her life, and for nearly twenty years afterward she was largely healthy, but her hearing slowly got worse, leading her to employ a series of hearing aids beginning in her late thirties. One day in 2000, at the age of forty-four, she woke up and found she couldn't hear out of her right ear. Getting out of bed, she fell flat on her face; her balance was gone as well. A spasm in the blood vessel that feeds the hair cells in the inner ear had starved them of oxygen, causing irreversible hearing loss. But her left ear, which had always been the "good" one, was unaffected. For three years she continued to be able to hear conversation, to enjoy music, and to function as a member of what is sometimes called the hearing world. We remained blissfully oblivious to the devastation that sudden, complete deafness could cause.

That ignorance ended abruptly that morning in June 2003. We had been packing boxes and preparing to drive to Waco to pick out a house. I was in the shower when I heard a sudden, desperate cry. "I can't hear anything!" Barbara exclaimed. Searching for something to say, I realized that nothing I could say would make any difference. Spoken words were futile. So I did what, as a Beethoven scholar, I knew Beethoven and his companions had done during the final decade of his life; I picked up a legal pad and began a "conversation book" in which I could write to her while she responded orally. We would fill dozens of them over the next several months.

There was a sublime coincidence in the fact that, having dedicated my life to the music of the world's most famous deaf musician, I now met deafness face to face. I had always known that Beethoven struggled with the most devastating handicap a musician could ever encounter. I also knew that he experienced profound social isolation during the last part of his life. I was intimately familiar with Beethoven's music, and I thought I understood his suffering. I had also known people who were hard of hearing and who had trouble in public spaces because background noise mixed indiscriminately with the sounds of conversation. But I had never spent significant time with someone who was profoundly deaf. That was about to change, and with it the whole trajectory of my life.

That devastating moment would be followed by a trip to the emergency room, where doctors injected steroids directly into

Barbara's inner ear in the hopes that they would stop and reverse the damage. We delayed our trip to Texas so that painful procedure could be repeated several times over the next few weeks. With the sobering realization that it was doing no good came fuller understanding that we had crossed a watershed in our life together and in that of our family. Never again, it seemed, would we be able to converse at the dinner table, watch television or a movie together, speak on the phone, or even exchange oral greetings. Conversation as we had always understood it was a thing of the past.

Barbara later said that the next six months, until modern technology came to our aid in the form of a cochlear implant in her left ear, felt like being in solitary confinement. Deafness, she imagined, was far worse than blindness could ever be. The latter simply deprives you of your ability to perceive the world. The former cuts you off from all contact with other human beings, placing you in a world seemingly beyond reach.

That was the world in which Beethoven lived out his final years, and like Barbara, he turned to technology for relief. Beethoven's surviving conversation books contain some discussion of an "electro vibrations machine" invented by a Dr. Carl Joseph Mayer in Vienna, although there is no indication that the famous composer ever submitted to such treatment.[1] He did make extensive use of ear trumpets for the magnification of sound, some of which were invented by his friend Johann Nepomuk Mälzel. He had a resonator built for his piano that may have allowed him to hear some sound even at the very end of his life. If cochlear implants had been available to him, I have little doubt that he would have gotten one, provided he was able to afford it.

The significance of these interventions has often been dismissed or minimized by those who have written about Beethoven. Nevertheless, it is unlikely he would have spent so much time experimenting with devices that did not yield results. Beethoven wanted to hear music better, and he also longed for human interaction. These are powerful motivators.

What Barbara and I learned over the eight and a half years of life that remained to her was that the adult human brain is more malleable than commonly believed, and even people with profound hearing loss can make surprising gains. Portions of the brain can be rededicated, and hearing can be at least partially relearned.

Shortly after we arrived at Baylor that August, an audiologist introduced us to the "pocket talker," a small box with an attached microphone that could transmit speech at high volume into a set of headphones. Before she began using this device, Barbara took a speech recognition test in a soundproof booth and scored only 3 percent with the residual hearing in her right ear. In the left she heard nothing at all. A few months later she took the same test and scored 40 or 50 percent. The physiology of her ear had not changed one iota. In the everyday world she still heard practically nothing; even the loud wail of a smoke alarm was barely audible. We had painstakingly practiced conversing, however. She eventually learned to understand much of what I said when I held the pocket talker at exactly the right angle and pitched my voice exactly right, and when she looked directly at me and read my lips to fill in the blanks. It was frustrating and it was slow. My words would blast from her headphones loudly enough to fill a whole room, and at first she still understood next to nothing. This was not an easy way to converse. Other than the conversation books, though, it was the only way, so we persisted. Those improved scores in the soundproof booth, achieved with no assistance from the pocket talker or lipreading, showed the result.

As for music, Barbara still heard nothing. Even over the headphones, it all sounded like a monotone. She was able to sing melodies that she already knew in reasonably good tune, due apparently to tactile memory in her vocal cords, but she could perceive no variation in pitch among the minimal sounds she was hearing. By improving her speech perception she had achieved one of Beethoven's goals, but the other one remained beyond her reach. If Barbara had lived in Beethoven's time, when only old-fashioned analog methods were available to amplify sound, that would probably have been the end of the story. But we knew there was an alternative, and we pursued it.

We had known about the existence of cochlear implants long before that fateful summer. The possibility that Barbara could be a candidate for one first came up when she lost the hearing in her right ear, but at that point insurance would not cover the expense because one working ear was considered sufficient. We also learned that scientists were experimenting with the regeneration of hair cells in the inner ear, which could conceivably cure the kind of hearing loss Barbara had experienced. An implant would have intruded on the cochlea and permanently destroyed that possibility. Once the left ear was gone, though, it didn't take long for a doctor to tell Barbara that a cochlear implant was in her future. Tests showed that her auditory nerve was in good condition, so it would convey signals to the hearing centers in the brain if those signals could be received. Shortly after moving to Texas we made contact with a physician at Baylor Medical Center in Dallas and began the process of moving toward implantation.

Let me acknowledge that this is a controversial procedure. In 2003, implants were already being given to very young children, as well as to adults who were prelingually deaf. Many in the Deaf community see this, justifiably, as a challenge to their identity: the latest in a series of attempts during recent history to discourage the use of American Sign Language and replace it with other, more "mainstream" ways of communicating. Those who don't support such efforts, known collectively as oralism, argue that deaf people will always be deaf—that that is a part of who they are, not a fault to be stigmatized and patched over with a high-tech fix that doesn't change the underlying condition. They understand themselves and others like them to be "big *D* deaf," meaning that deafness is a part of their cultural identity.

Barbara, though, was not used to thinking of herself as deaf. She knew no ASL and had no deaf friends. Much of her enjoyment in life, and of our life together, was based on hearing and participating in music. There was no question in either of our minds that a procedure that promised to restore even a portion of her hearing was a miracle to be embraced. We met with other adult implant recipients and found that many of them could carry on conversations with considerable fluency, and some could enjoy and even perform music. Our insurance approved the procedure, which would have been beyond our financial reach otherwise. Shortly before Thanksgiving 2003, an incision was made behind Barbara's left ear, a hole was drilled in her skull to accommodate the implant, and an array of electrodes was attached to her cochlea. The implant included a metal plate under her skin, which would later allow an external processor to be connected with a magnet. She was sent home to recuperate, still hearing next to nothing.

Activation was scheduled for my birthday, December 19. We drove the hundred miles back to Dallas with a mix of hope and dread. There was no guarantee it would work at all. If it did, we had no idea how well it would work or whether the sounds would be recognizable. We understood that Barbara would have to learn to hear once again as an adult.

At activation she was given an external processor resembling a large hearing aid that fit behind her left ear. A magnet, which she placed on her head, attached itself to the implant through a loose connection that could easily be broken by a sudden movement or touch. The device was powered by a battery that carried enough charge to run it for about four hours; a collection of three spares had to be kept charged and ready to replace it when it ran out of power, which happened without warning. On that first visit and at subsequent "mappings" (they continued monthly for most of that first year), the implant was connected to a computer and a host of adjustments were made to the signal based on her response to auditory cues. When the audiologist was satisfied that we were doing as well as possible—I at speaking to her, she at hearing what I said—she sent us home and told us not to use the pocket talker anymore. The goal now was to adjust to hearing with the implant.

Viral videos have shown both adults and children reacting to activation with wonder and delight. Our experience was more earthbound. When the first sounds—just isolated tones— were transmitted from the audiologist's computer to Barbara's implant, her face didn't change. I found myself straining to imagine what she was experiencing, since for anyone else there was no sound to hear; all that registered was bars on the computer screen. Moments later, when the implant's internal microphone was allowed to kick in, things didn't improve. Barbara appeared disoriented and a bit frightened by the way my voice sounded inside her head. It was a bittersweet moment. The fear that the implant wouldn't work, which I had hardly dared acknowledge during all the preliminaries, gave way to a dread both gentler and more deep-seated. I knew now that she could hear me through the tangle of circuitry that pressed on her skull both inside and out. I could also see how hard she was working to make these strange electronic bursts congeal into words and sentences. I sensed that that quest, with its trials and exhilarations, would become the central fact of her life, and would define the nature and quality of our togetherness. The drive back to Waco did not bode well. Barbara could not understand me nearly as well as she had been able to with the pocket talker. I sounded, she said, like a squawking cartoon character. Since it was my birthday we went out to dinner, but the mood was more subdued than celebratory. We were both exhausted from the anticipation. We went to bed that night still not knowing what to expect.

Over the weeks and months that followed, I grew more hopeful as I watched Barbara gradually adjust to the information she was receiving through her previously useless left auditory nerve. My voice moved down in pitch and began to sound more like what she remembered. We deliberately sought out loud public places in which to practice talking to each other, and her comprehension increased substantially. We took walks and she tried to recognize the sounds she was hearing. One of the most instructive moments occurred when a dog barked. "What was that?" Barbara asked. I said, "A dog barking." The next time she heard it, later on the same walk, it actually sounded like a dog barking to her. She said the experience resembled going through a giant Rolodex in her brain and pulling up sound memories to associate with the auditory input she was now receiving. Once the association had been made, the learning process appeared to be entirely passive. If she knew what it was she was hearing, it sounded the way it was supposed to. If she didn't, it didn't. It was as simple, and as bafflingly elusive, as that.

A breakthrough moment occurred a few months later as she was listening to the car radio. She had been leaving it on as she drove around town, tuned to a top-forty station, in the hope that she would recognize something, but so far everything had sounded the same: like a station with very bad reception from which only occasional glimmers of recognizable music emerged. Suddenly she found she understood the words "eight days a week." From that point on the Beatles song "clicked" into place, and she heard the rest of it just as she remembered it sounding. The Rolodex had yielded another hit.

As I observed these things, I gained new, if vague, insights into the ways in which the human brain recognizes auditory signals and learns to connect them with the reservoir formed by past experience. I realized that such connections are always forming anew and that they can take surprising shapes and exponential leaps. I also realized that Beethoven, with his ear trumpets, his resonator, and his vast musical training, must have had such experiences too. The familiar narrative of a musician gradually, inexorably losing his hearing and coming to terms with the loss in his creative work was a compelling one, but it couldn't be the whole story.

In this book I can't claim to be telling the whole story either. What I do hope to do is make new connections based on three interrelated sources: my own musical training, my knowledge of Beethoven's biography and his creative life, and my personal experience watching my wife lose and partially regain her hearing. This is a story nobody else could tell. I hope my telling of it will be ear-opening for anyone intrigued by the human heart, the human mind, and the mysterious harmony that binds them together.

* 1 *
Beethoven's Deafness

WHAT WE KNOW,
WHAT WE CAN ONLY GUESS

Hearing loss sneaks up on you. Its first symptoms are often subtle and easily explained away—especially if you're a musician who takes pride in the acuity of your hearing. "Having a good ear" is a familiar metaphor for having musical talent. If one day a friend's speech is a bit difficult to understand, or a sound heard by someone else fails to register, it is easy and tempting to blame it on something other than deafness. Yet the fact is that musicians are more prone to lose their hearing than most other people. Hours spent practicing in small rooms or playing with large ensembles can take their toll, and it is not unusual for an experienced musician to begin to suspect that his or her ears aren't as good as they used to be. The high rate of hearing loss among musicians, classical as well as popular, is a well-kept professional secret, because denial of the condition starts with musicians themselves. Many simply don't want to admit they have a problem.[1]

One can only imagine, therefore, how early Ludwig van Beethoven began to notice that his ears were betraying him. What we do know is when he found it impossible to remain in denial. On June 29, 1801, the thirty-year-old composer wrote a letter to an old friend from Bonn, Dr. Franz Wegeler, which is often cited but nevertheless worth quoting at length.[2] After a short summary of his present circumstances, Beethoven wrote that despite his professional success, "that jealous demon, my poor health, has played a nasty trick on me. To wit, for three years my hearing has become steadily weaker. This supposedly stems from my lower abdomen, which, as you know, has long given me distress, but has grown worse here." A local doctor had prescribed treatments both for the intestinal symptoms he described and for his ears, and while the former had been successful,

> my ears continue to ring and hiss day and night. I must say that I lead a wretched life. For two years I have avoided nearly all company, since it is impossible for me to tell people that I am deaf.... To give you an idea of this strange deafness, let me tell you that at the theater I must lean in very near to the orchestra in order to understand the actor. If I am some distance away, I do not hear the higher notes of instruments and voices. I am surprised that there are people who have never noticed it in conversation; since I am often distracted, they attribute it to that. Much of the time I can hardly hear someone who speaks quietly—the sounds perhaps, but not the words—but as soon as someone shouts I find it unbearable.[3]

Beethoven went on to say that one of his doctors had assured him that his hearing would get better, although it would never be fully restored.

One thing that is clear from this letter is that physicians of Beethoven's time—presumably including Wegeler, to whom he described his symptoms in detail—had little understanding of the causes and treatment of hearing loss. Neither they nor the composer seems to have questioned the assumption that his growing deafness was connected to his long-standing digestive symptoms. One doctor treated his ears with almond oil, while another prescribed baths in the Danube for both conditions. Not surprisingly, neither treatment helped him to hear better.

With the benefit of hindsight, it is also evident that Beethoven had at least two symptoms widely associated with sensorineural hearing loss, one of the two major types of deafness recognized by today's doctors. Unlike conductive hearing loss, which results when sounds are blocked from reaching the inner ear, sensorineural hearing loss stems from malfunctions in the inner ear itself, where the sense of hearing is centered, or in the nerves that transmit its signals to the brain. The symptoms Beethoven experienced reflect not just an absence of sound but distortions in the way he perceived it: tinnitus ("ringing in the ears") is an annoying, often maddening auditory illusion characterized by persistent sounds that seem to originate inside the victim's head; the unbearably loud shouting, or "loudness recruitment," occurs when the brain compensates for a loss of auditory information at low volumes by registering sounds of greater intensity as being louder than they actually are.[4] If Beethoven began to notice these symptoms at twenty-seven, it is likely that the process that produced them began even earlier.

What caused these symptoms to develop in a man in his mid-twenties? We may never know for sure, because Beethoven's temporal bones, including the bones of the inner ears, were removed during his autopsy and have since disappeared. Still, we can make some reasoned speculations. Deafness from sensorineural causes can manifest suddenly and with no warning, but it can also develop gradually, either as a result of aging or due to external causes. Excessive exposure to loud sounds often plays a major role, but viral infections can contribute as well, as can circulatory problems that interfere with the supply of blood to the inner ear.

In Beethoven's case, two possible explanations have been advanced for the onset of his condition. He is said to have become seriously sick during the summer of 1796; the illness, according to one source, "settled in his organs of hearing, and from this time on his deafness steadily increased."[5] While the fact of such an illness is accepted by Beethoven's most celebrated biographer,[6] its exact date and nature are unknown. Beethoven is also said to have had an episode of typhoid fever during his youth, which could possibly have resulted in nerve damage.[7]

Beethoven himself is said to have suggested a different explanation to his English friend Charles Neate. As a young man, he said, he was working on an opera (not *Fidelio*) and had to deal with a very difficult tenor: hearing a knock at his door, he reportedly said, "I sprang up from my table under such an excitement of rage that, as the man entered the room, I threw myself upon the floor as they do upon the stage, coming down upon my hands. When I arose I found myself deaf and have been so ever since. The physicians say the nerve is injured."[8] This account is suspicious for several reasons; it is reported thirdhand and well after the event,[9] and the statement that Beethoven was deaf from that point forward is inconsistent with accounts of a gradual hearing loss. It should be noted, though, that while *Fidelio* was Beethoven's only complete opera, he probably wrote a tenor solo for Ignaz Umlauf's *Die schöne Schusterin* in or around 1796,[10] which is the same year he later claimed his deafness began. The author of an essay on Beethoven's medical history notes that "this would describe an attack of vertigo, 'labyrinthine apoplexy,' from interference with the blood supply to or bleeding in the auditory region."[11] This is also the only time Beethoven is said to have reported symptoms resembling the dizziness that is frequently associated with inner-ear disease; as the same author points out, the reflexive "threw myself" can be understood as a passive construction and doesn't mean that the fall was deliberate.[12]

By documentary standards, neither of these stories is satisfactory, and they could easily be dismissed as mere rumor or speculation. It is certainly possible, though, that Beethoven suffered the beginning of hearing loss around 1796 due either to a recent or past physical illness or to a vascular episode in which his inner ears were temporarily deprived of blood. These are now, and were then, among the most common causes of sensorineural deafness.

As I have already noted, there is an entirely different category of hearing loss that results from conductivity problems inside the ear. These may also result from infection, or even from a simple accumulation of earwax. Conductive hearing loss, though, may also be caused by otosclerosis, or abnormal growth of the bones that lie in the middle ear between the eardrum and the cochlea. These include the ossicles, or "little bones": the malleus, the incus, and the stapes, also known as the hammer, the anvil, and the stirrup. If these lose their flexibility and cannot move, sound vibrations cannot travel past the eardrum. Otosclerosis is a hereditary condition, and the fact that nobody else in Beethoven's family is reported to have suffered from it makes this diagnosis problematic. However, it may also be activated by viral infections, including common diseases like measles that Beethoven might well have experienced.[13] (Though Beethoven bore on his face the scars of smallpox, measles was so commonplace that it was unlikely to have been mentioned in the historical record.) In simple conductive hearing loss, the auditory nerves, including the hair cells in the cochlea, are not affected; rather, external sounds are blocked before they can reach them.

It has long been suggested that the nature and progress of Beethoven's deafness, along with the time in his life when his symptoms began to appear, are consistent with a diagnosis of cochlear otosclerosis, which straddles the two categories.[14] In this condition, hardening takes place in the cochlear endosteum: the connective tissue between the stapes and the cochlea. In many cases this leads to fixation of the stapes; the stirrup, the closest bone to the inner ear, becomes immobile, so vibrations cannot be transmitted to the cochlea. Even when this fixation does not occur, cochlear otosclerosis is often associated with damage to the hair cells of the cochlea and the auditory nerve, which connects the inner ear with the brain, resulting in sensorineural hearing loss.[15] Whether Beethoven's stapes were fixed in this manner may never be known, since the doctor who performed his autopsy did not comment. The autopsy did confirm damage to his auditory nerves, however. Taken in connection with Beethoven's observed symptoms, this establishes beyond a reasonable doubt that his deafness was at least in part sensorineural. The most common hypothesis is that his stapes were also fixed, resulting in mixed sensorineural and conductive hearing loss. Such a diagnosis would be consistent with all the symptoms Beethoven and others reported, and cochlear otosclerosis is a likely cause.[16] This might have been triggered by one of Beethoven's numerous illnesses, and it does not rule out the possibility of labyrinthine apoplexy or other contributing factors.[17]

Needless to say, with a case as famous as Beethoven's a provisional diagnosis like this is subject to challenge, and many other hypotheses have also been put forth. A series of writers from Romain Rolland through Maynard Solomon have argued that Beethoven's deafness was at least to some extent self-inflicted; Rolland blamed it on the "furious concentration" that characterized Beethoven's genius, whose effects he compared to those of yogic meditation, and Solomon suggested that it fulfilled a psychological need.[18] Beethoven's deafness has been blamed on syphilis, although there is no proof he had the disease.[19] It has been blamed on alcoholism, although there is no proof he was an alcoholic and no obvious reason this would have caused him to become deaf.[20] Most recently, there was a flurry of attention to claims that Beethoven suffered from plumbism, or lead poisoning, caused either by medical malpractice during his final illness or by a lifelong habit of drinking cheap wine.[21] There actually is a possibility that an inflammation of the bowel could also damage the ears, but the symptoms of such an inflammation do not seem to match those that Beethoven reported.[22] Nevertheless, an argument has been made that autoimmune bowel disease is the most persuasive explanation for Beethoven's deafness.[23] He certainly suffered from severe intestinal problems throughout his adult life, so it is at least worth considering that his two most notable health problems were in some way related.[24]

While Beethoven's hearing loss is often described as gradual and inexorable, it appears likely that for more than ten years after the letter to Wegeler there was actually little change. In 1802 Beethoven's friends began noticing his deafness, although they may well have suspected it earlier and kept it to themselves. The first written description is provided by Ferdinand Ries, and it is searing in its directness. He and Beethoven were walking in the fields around Heiligenstadt, a country town outside Vienna where Beethoven's doctor had sent him to rest his hearing, and where the Heiligenstadt Testament would be written a few months later: the document in which he poured out his heart to his brothers about his increasing emotional distress. Hearing a shepherd playing on a wooden flute, Ries remarked on it to Beethoven, who was forced to admit that he heard nothing.[25] The ruse could no longer be maintained. There is another version of this story, though, also from Ries, that describes a similar incident a few years later.[26] Since Beethoven alludes to the flute incident in the Heiligenstadt Testament, the earlier story is probably true, but the later one suggests that little changed in the ensuing years; he could still pretend he was fooling people until directly confronted with evidence to the contrary.

In 1804, when he was thirty-three years old, Beethoven is said to have had trouble hearing the wind instruments when the full orchestra was playing at rehearsals for the recently completed *Eroica* Symphony, but the letter to Wegeler ("if I am some distance away I do not hear the higher notes of instruments and voices") suggests that this would have been true three years earlier as well. In 1808, at the nearly interminable concert at which both the Fifth and Sixth Symphonies were premiered, Beethoven stopped the orchestra in the middle of his Fantasy for Piano, Chorus, and Orchestra, op. 80, because of a breakdown in the orchestral accompaniment. This occurred at a point at which only two oboes are supposed to be playing with the piano, and according to an eyewitness account the clarinets entered at the same time, sixteen measures early. Beethoven tried to stop the clarinets and apparently succeeded, but was so dissatisfied that he forced the orchestra to start again from the beginning.[27] Since only a few instruments were playing, this account does not contradict the report from 1804. The oboe and clarinet parts in question, though, are harmonically fairly similar, and Beethoven could have let the mistake pass. The fact that it disturbed him enough to cause him to stop a performance in progress shows that his hearing of live music was still suprisingly accurate.

Perhaps more significantly, early the next year he sent some minor corrections to his publisher Breitkopf und Härtel based on having heard the symphonies in performance. "When I gave them to you," he wrote, "I had not yet heard any part of them, and one must not try to be so godlike as not to try to improve anything here and there in one's creations."[28] The primary musical change comes at the beginning of the second movement of the *Pastoral* Symphony, the "Scene by the Brook," and it is subtle but significant. The movement opens with a fragmentary melody in the first violins backed up by a rocking accompaniment in 12/8 meter by the second violins, violas, and cellos, all playing with mutes. The manuscript divides the entire cello section into two groups, indicated by the fact that Beethoven wrote two separate parts on a single staff. In the second letter to his publisher, Beethoven specified that these parts should be played by two solo cellos and that the rest of the cellos should play with the basses, as was often the case in orchestral music at the time.[29] This change required a sophisticated judgment about the sonic balance of an ensemble that at times has up to six distinct harmonic parts, and Beethoven apparently made it either after hearing the music performed or, more likely, during rehearsal.[30]

Until at least 1812 Beethoven also carried on conversations successfully enough to have an active, if limited, social life and several love affairs; the ear trumpets and conversation books came later. Thus while his hearing does appear to have deteriorated quickly during the 1810s, for a dozen or so years before that he was hardly the deaf musician of popular conception. In May 1809 he was so distressed by the noise of Napoleon's bombardment of Vienna that he buried his head in pillows in the cellar of his brother Caspar Carl's house. This suggests that his loudness recruitment was still active enough to produce acute discomfort—the same kind of discomfort that he reported to Wegeler in 1801 when people spoke too loudly.

A letter written to Wegeler on May 2, 1810, is revealing. Beethoven said that he would be happy, "perhaps one of the happiest of people, if the demon had not taken up residence in my ears. If I had not read somewhere that one should not willingly depart from this life as long as he can accomplish something worthwhile, I would be long gone, and by my own hand. Life is so beautiful, but for me it is poisoned forever."[31] Reading this, it is natural to assume that Beethoven is referring to his deafness. The wording, though, is actively affirmative—"wenn nicht der Dämon in meinen Ohren seinen Aufenthalt aufgeschlagen"— suggesting a malicious presence rather than an absence. It is possible that the demon in his ears was not deafness but tinnitus; despite its popular description as "ringing in the ears," this affliction can in fact be so devastatingly loud as to drive a person near madness. As we have seen, Beethoven complained about this already in 1801.

It was probably in 1811 or 1812 that Beethoven noted on a page of what has come to be called the Petter sketchbook that "cotton in my ears at the pianoforte frees my hearing from the disagreeable noise."[32] Beethoven's wording here is ambiguous; *das unangenehm Rauschende* could signify anything from rustling to thunderous roaring. Given that Beethoven sought to be free from it, though, it is more likely that it was at the louder end of this range. The fact that he felt particular discomfort when playing the piano is consistent with the experience of other musicians with hearing loss and loudness recruitment. The problem is not that they can't hear but that they hear too much, so that playing—particularly at a percussive instrument like the piano—can be agonizing. Beethoven dealt with this by putting cotton in his ears. More recent sufferers have used earplugs. As we will see in chapter 5, this strategy can backfire, augmenting the loudness recruitment and perhaps accelerating the progress of the underlying deafness. This may very well be why Beethoven's hearing began to deteriorate more rapidly after 1810.

There are multiple witnesses who claim that Beethoven's hearing loss initially fluctuated rather than steadily advancing. Ries claimed that in the early years it entirely disappeared for a time.[33] Andreas Wawruch, his doctor during his final years, reported that "when he entered his 30th year, he developed a hemorrhoid condition together with an annoying noise and ringing in both ears. Soon he became hard of hearing and, although he experienced periods of remission that could last several months, his ailment finally led to total deafness."[34] Like so much else, these stories are anecdotal, and it is hard to know whether they can be trusted. In his surviving letters Beethoven makes no reference to any improvement or remission. The most likely cause of fluctuating sensorineural hearing loss would be Ménière's disease, a condition caused by fluid buildup in the inner ears. However, this almost always involves severe episodes of dizziness, which Beethoven is not reported to have experienced.[35] In the absence of more definite evidence, therefore, we should probably not assume that Beethoven's hearing varied to any great degree later in his life — something that in any case is suggested neither by Ries nor by Wawruch and is only hinted at by a few later sources.[36] He may well have had a harder time hearing in louder or less acoustically congenial environments, or when he was excessively tired or under stress. He certainly would have found it easier to understand the voices of people with whom he conversed regularly. Some voices may simply have lain primarily within the range where his residual hearing was best, while others lay primarily outside of it. All of this is consistent with the experience of other people with hearing loss.[37]

✺

Clearly there is not enough evidence to reach a conclusive diagnosis of the cause of Beethoven's deafness; all we can do is examine its effects and speculate. Before we turn to the decline of his hearing during the final fifteen years of his life, it is worth pausing to take stock of the personal and emotional toll these early symptoms caused him. One curious fact that emerges from the 1801 letter to Wegeler is that Beethoven did not seem overly concerned about his future as a musician. He said that if he were in another line of work deafness would be less of a problem, but what he mostly meant was that his enemies—of whom he claimed to have many—would have a field day if they found out. He said nothing about how the problem was affecting his dual careers as a piano virtuoso, in which capacity he was in high demand, and as a composer; in fact, he anticipated a future visit to Bonn during which he would be able to perform for the benefit of the poor.

This point is largely borne out by a letter that he wrote to his friend Carl Amenda two days later, on July 1. "Know that the thing I value most, my hearing, has much deteriorated," he told Amenda. "I already felt traces of this when you were with me [Amenda had left Vienna in the fall of 1799] but said nothing. Now it is getting continually worse, and it remains to be seen whether it can be made well again."[38] Beethoven expressed concern that his best years would go by without his being able to accomplish everything that he might have, but he went on to say that "my ailment bothers me least when I am playing and composing, and is at its worst in company." His piano playing, he said, had improved considerably.[39]

What mostly concerned him was the social isolation that poor hearing inevitably entails. In another letter to Wegeler dated November 16, 1801, he said that for the past two years he had shunned human society and must appear to be a misanthrope. Less than a year later, in October 1802, he penned the Heiligenstadt Testament, addressed to his brothers Carl and Johann.[40] "Oh you people who take me for hostile, obstinate, or misanthropic," he wrote, seemingly speaking to humankind at large, "you do me a great injustice. You do not know the secret of what makes me appear that way. . . . Just consider that for six years I have been beset by an incurable condition, made worse by ignorant doctors, deceived year after year into hoping for improvement, and am finally compelled to face the prospect of a lasting malady (from which recovery may take years or may even be impossible)."[41] He went on to confirm what he had written to Amenda: that his deafness had caused him to isolate himself socially, and that as a musician it was particularly painful for him to acknowledge his affliction.

It is remarkable that nowhere in the document did Beethoven express concern about the future of his professional life. In fact, he said that it was only the thought of all the creative work he had yet to do that had held him back from suicide. The pain he expressed was due solely to the fact that he had felt compelled to avoid human society, both because of the difficulty in communicating and because of the embarrassment he feared experiencing when he was identified as a deaf musician. The statement that this had been going on for six years pushes the origins of his deafness back until at least 1796. This was also the year that Beethoven had last seen Franz Wegeler in person.[42] Wegeler, whose early biographical sketch of the composer was structured around their correspondence, quotes a letter he received from their mutual friend Stephan von Breuning, dated October 13, 1804, when Breuning was sharing an apartment with Beethoven. "You would not believe, dear Wegeler, what an indescribable and, I should say, truly dreadful impact the loss of his hearing has had on him. Imagine the feeling of being unhappy—and with such a vehement nature as his. Add to this his shyness, distrust (often of his best friends) and general indecisiveness! For the most part, except for the occasional moments when his original affection expresses itself freely, association with him is a real strain, and one can never be quite off one's guard."[43]

It is clear that Beethoven was suffering, that he was acutely self-conscious, and that his status as a musician with poor hearing was a source of paralyzing embarrassment to him. What is less clear is the extent to which his condition bothered him musically. This statement is so strongly counterintuitive that it needs to be drawn out and examined further. There is a presumption in the Beethoven literature that the composer was depressed over his growing deafness primarily because his hearing was his most valuable professional asset. Of course, for someone so heavily invested in music this would have been a strong personal loss as well. One might expect Beethoven to have said in his letters, "I am tormented by the thought that I will never again be able to hear music performed with the enjoyment it has given me in the past," or "I never sit down at the piano without contrasting my present poor hearing with the way things sounded when I was a young man." Most of all, one might expect him to be in despair at the thought of not being able to hear his own music and to be deterred from composing by this prospect. For years Beethoven had been in the habit of improvising at the piano and writing down his ideas in the form of sketches, which he later transformed into finished compositions. He might well have worried about whether he could continue to work in this manner.

Instead his anguish had to do almost entirely with the way his relationships with others had deteriorated, with the unjust judgments he believed others were making about him personally, and with the tormenting noises in his ears. It was at this very point that he resolved to put new energy into his work as a composer: one who would continue to play and conduct in public, if only sporadically, for more than another decade.[44]

And how did his despair over his growing deafness affect his music? During the Heiligenstadt crisis in 1802, his main project was the sunny, comical Second Symphony, which has led to the suggestion that he used that work as a vehicle of escape. Three symphonies later, of course, he created a powerful and enduring four-note symbol of defiance. "So klopft das Schicksaal an die Pforte," his notably unreliable biographer Anton Schindler reported that he said of the Fifth Symphony's opening motive: a comment that, if correctly translated, means that fate is pounding at the gate. Perhaps the most autobiographical moment in his music, though, came at the beginning of the final act (the second in the version we know today) of his opera *Fidelio*, first performed in 1805. The hero Florestan, bound in chains and cast into solitary confinement in an underground dungeon, first appears nearly dead from starvation, victim of an arbitrary vendetta. In a line of melody that also appears near the beginning of the second and third *Leonore* overtures—the latter among the most powerful instrumental works Beethoven created—Florestan laments that in the springtime of his life, his happiness has been taken from him. Cut off from all human contact, he finds that everything he values is gone and may never be restored. It is probably no coincidence that when Beethoven revised this opera in 1814, his deafness and social isolation now closing in with tyrannical force, he lavished more attention on this scene than on any other. The powerful instrumental introduction draws the audience directly into the depths of Florestan's soul, laying Beethoven's bare as well.

By 1814 Beethoven indeed had reason to despair. Two years before, his most serious attempt to find lasting love with a woman had ended unhappily, its only surviving trace the "Immortal Beloved" letter of July 6 and 7, 1812, in which he poured out his heart to the apparent love of his life while simultaneously ending their relationship. After years of relative stability, his hearing was now in rapid decline, making it more unlikely than ever that he would find love and domestic happiness. His fame and professional success were perhaps at their all-time high during his lifetime, but this must have rung ironically hollow.

Numerous witnesses testify that conversation with the composer was becoming more and more difficult. After 1812 he began to make use of ear trumpets designed by his friend Johann Nepomuk Mälzel (1772–1838): lengths of tubing whose hollow end could be inserted into his ear and which rapidly expanded, in some cases leading to a resonating device to pick up sound. These were essentially inverted megaphones and as such worked much like later hearing aids, providing an amplified sound stream that was fed directly into Beethoven's ear canal. After 1812, attempts to communicate with Beethoven often involved a lot of shouting and embarrassment, as can be the case today with people with hearing loss. He seems not to have recognized when his voice was too loud,[45] a problem familiar to those who often converse with the postlingually deaf. His piano playing became intolerable to listen to; according to Louis Spohr, who heard him rehearse the *Archduke* Trio, op. 97, in 1814, he often missed notes and didn't seem to care that the piano was out of tune.[46] His final public performance at the piano took place on January 25, 1815, accompanying Franz Wild in his song "Adelaide,"[47] and around this time he also began to need an assistant when conducting. All of this suggests that his hearing was rapidly deteriorating and that he was struggling to adjust.

Perhaps most significant of all, Beethoven composed little music during the years between 1812 and 1818, especially if his output is judged by the prodigious standards of the preceding decade.[48] This lapse in creativity has been attributed to various causes. The "heroic" style of his middle period, ushered in by the *Eroica* Symphony in 1803, had perhaps run its course. The fall of Napoleon and the reactionary Metternich regime that followed supposedly marked the end of the political optimism and hope in progress that had spurred the imaginations of Beethoven and his peers. The end of the "Immortal Beloved" affair may have left Beethoven deeply depressed.

Here, though, the irony noted earlier is turned on its head; few people seem to have given much weight to the possibility that as his hearing went into its final decline, Beethoven began to doubt whether he could continue composing at all, and that this was the main reason for his depression and lack of creativity during these years.

Such doubts would have attacked him from several fronts. For a creative person the loss of a crucial skill or asset is devastating in itself, and Beethoven in these years found he was no longer able to function as a pianist, as a conductor, or as a listener. Like most highly trained musicians, he would still have been able to look at a score and imagine the sounds in his head. This, however, is in no way a substitute for actually hearing music performed. An essential part of music making comes from the interaction between the performer and the notes; it is the performer's musical personality that transforms the written record into a living and meaningful experience of sound. To lose this is to lose both music and the social experience that music has always been. Even to sit down by oneself at a piano and play is to apply one's own musical substance to the task and embark on a voyage of discovery. And Beethoven was accustomed not just to playing scores but to improvising: to creating music on the fly by fusing himself with the stubborn and resistant keyboard and pushing it to, and often beyond, its limits. Doing so in public was the ultimate demonstration of his mastery of the medium, and it required live listeners to provide a feedback loop and spur him on. Doing so in private was his preferred method of composing, and we can only guess at the

extent to which his written sketches and often chaotic manuscripts fed both off and into live improvisation. What is clear
is that he was his own most critical and inspirational listener.
He was now losing that listener, in a way that had probably still
been unimaginable at the time of the Heiligenstadt Testament.

Beethoven's loss was also no doubt a severe blow to his personal identity. Modern psychology provides some helpful insights into how that identity was formed and maintained. Beethoven's father, a severe alcoholic, sought very early to exploit
his son's exceptional talent, and it is reasonable to assume that
the results plagued the son for the rest of his life. The most obvious manifestation of this was the fact that he remained confused about his actual age, since his father had represented him
as being two years younger than he was in the hopes of present-
ing him as a Mozartian child prodigy. Like Mozart, therefore,
Beethoven grew up understanding that he existed to serve his
father's emotional needs and to bolster his father's self-image,
rather than the other way around. He was the prototypical
"gifted child," and like most in his position he also grew accustomed to seeking validation through public recognition of his
talent. In her path-breaking book *The Drama of the Gifted Child*,
psychoanalyst Alice Miller described the profile of a narcissis-
tically disturbed patient in terms that can easily by applied to
Beethoven:

> Quite often we are faced here with gifted patients who
> have been praised and admired for their talents and their
> achievements. . . . According to prevailing, general atti-
> tudes, these people—the pride of their parents—should
> have had a strong and stable sense of self-assurance. But ex-
> actly the opposite is the case. In everything they undertake
> they do well and often excellently; they are admired and
> envied; they are successful whenever they care to be—but

all to no avail. Behind all this lurks depression, the feeling of emptiness and self-alienation, and a sense that their
life has no meaning. These dark feelings will come to the
fore as soon as the drug of grandiosity fails, as soon as they
are not "on top," not definitely the "superstar," or whenever they suddenly get the feeling they failed to live up to
some ideal image and measure they feel they must adhere
to. Then they are plagued by anxiety or deep feelings of
guilt and shame.[49]

In the Heiligenstadt Testament, Beethoven was clearly struggling to construct a sense of self-worth based on his continued
ability to compose, despite the humiliation caused by his failing hearing which he described in the 1801 letter to Wegeler. If
by 1812 he was once again doubting that ability, this would be
more than sufficient to explain the depths of depression that
he suffered during the ensuing years. As Miller points out, such
people often reach to their own children for validation, thus
perpetuating the cycle. Beethoven had no child of his own, so
it is hardly surprising that he now devoted a great deal of his energy to seeking one, rather than to the increasingly challenging
task of composing music.

⁀

The saga of Beethoven's desperate struggle to gain custody of
his nephew Karl after his brother Caspar Carl's death in 1815
is rightly seen as a blot on his biography, and perhaps as evidence of a defect in his character. In light of his growing deafness, though—the manifest failure of his effort to live up to
the ideal image of a musician—it was also utterly predictable.
For the next few years he may have devoted more time to trying to wrest Karl away from his mother Johanna than he did to

writing music. In this attempt he finally succeeded. As is well known, Karl, buffeted about between his admittedly dissolute mother and his eccentric, increasingly deaf uncle, grew into an emotionally confused young man who attempted suicide in 1826. What is less well understood is that by attaching himself to Karl as he did, Beethoven probably once again constructed a reason to go on living.

Having done so, he could then return to the challenge of composing from somewhat firmer ground. Most of the great works of the late period, including the Ninth Symphony and the *Missa Solemnis*, the final piano sonatas and string quartets, and the Diabelli variations, were substantially written during the last decade of Beethoven's life, when his deafness had progressed to the point that he could no longer perform in public and others had to communicate with him largely in writing. This is still not a large output compared to what Beethoven had produced during similar periods earlier in his life, and his working method seems to have been even more deliberate than ever. Despite some feverish bursts of activity and a large number of minor works written to make money, Beethoven produced barely over one major piece a year during this time. Nevertheless, these are among the most widely admired and respected compositions in the entire history of music. Beethoven's deafness may have slowed him down, but it also led to works of unsurpassed profundity.

How did Beethoven create music at such a high level when he was unable to hear it? This is a mystery that may never be solved, but it is nonetheless a mystery worth explaining. Simply to say that he remembered the sounds of music and imagined them in his head is to evade it, not to answer it. But it is also possible that Beethoven was never actually entirely deaf. In fact, George Thomas Ealy, in a pathbreaking article published in 1994, went so far as to suggest that "the commonly held belief that Beethoven was functionally deaf should be dismissed. . . .

His late works were not composed in complete deafness but in a state of limited hearing."[50]

Ealy devoted several pages to reviewing the evidence about Beethoven's hearing during the last years of his life, which is mostly anecdotal and often contradictory. Strangely, after pouring out his heart in the letters to Amenda and others and in the Heiligenstadt Testament, during this time Beethoven himself had little to say about his deafness, even though the volume of his surviving correspondence is considerably higher. For one thing, the cat was out of the bag—the *Allgemeine musikalische Zeitung*, the most widely read periodical in the German-speaking musical world, first reported his deafness in 1816, and by the time he died it was clearly common knowledge.[51] There are reports, though, of his improvising in private with great success late in his life, even though others found his playing to be a pale echo of what it had been.[52] While he began using conversation books in 1818 when speaking with people in public, and an erasable tablet at home, there are suggestions that he could still understand speech well beyond this point.[53] He kept sketchpads on a table next to his piano as late as 1826 (the last year in which he composed anything).[54] He also used a resonator built by the Viennese piano manufacturer Matthäus Andreas Stein to fit over his Broadwood piano, installed in the late summer of 1820; this was important enough to him that when the Viennese Graf piano firm loaned him a piano in 1826, they manufactured a similar device to go with it.[55]

One myth about Beethoven's hearing during the last years probably needs to be discarded. At the 1824 premiere of the Ninth Symphony he is often described as continuing to mark time, his head lost in the score, after the performance was over. Contralto Karoline Unger then had to turn the oblivious composer around in order to alert him to the cheers of the audience. This image of a distracted Beethoven immersed in his own world could not contrast more strongly with a description written later that year by Friedrich August Kanne, who witnessed both the premiere and the repeat performance a few weeks later. Kanne described "the transfigured master at the side of the directing Capellmeister Umlauf, reading along in the score, feeling doubly every small nuance and gradation of delivery and almost indicating them."[56] This depiction of Beethoven as minutely attentive to the details of the performance accords with other written accounts from the last years of his life. Violinist Joseph Böhm, for example, described rehearsing the String Quartet in E-flat Major, op. 127, in Beethoven's presence the year after the Ninth Symphony premiere: "It was studied industriously and rehearsed frequently under Beethoven's own eyes: I said Beethoven's *eyes* intentionally, for the unhappy man was so deaf that he could no longer hear the heavenly sound of his compositions. And yet rehearsing in his presence was not easy. With close attention his eyes followed the bows and therefore he was able to judge the smallest fluctuations in tempo or rhythm and correct them immediately."[57]

Kanne and Böhm thus lend support to the alternative story that Unger turned Beethoven around at the conclusion of the scherzo, not at that of the finale. By this account Beethoven would have been aware that the music, which was within his line of sight, had stopped, but unaware that the audience, which was behind him, was on its feet applauding: something that would not have been unusual for an audience at the time after a dynamic and exciting movement like this one. His sensitivity to sound, in other words, was minimal, even though his awareness of music remained surprisingly acute.

⁕

As to how Beethoven composed during his final years, while it may be unwise to speculate too broadly based on his finished works, there is a passage in the Piano Sonata in A-flat Major, op. 110, written in 1821, that might provide a glimpse. The sonata concludes with an extraordinary fusion of a slow arioso—a lyrical, songlike passage—and a faster fugue. This section is introduced by a rhapsodic, improvisatory opening that lacks a time signature in the traditional sense. After the fugue runs its course, the arioso is repeated a half step lower, with added pauses and ornaments that also convey the urgency of improvisation. Then, for three extraordinary measures,[58] Beethoven writes a widely spaced G major chord, separated by rests, ten times in a row, with only two changes in voicing. It begins at the default dynamic level of *piano* and crescendos, with both the damper and *una corda* pedals held down, to an unspecified louder volume, after which a diminuendo leads to another fugue based on an inversion of the initial subject (example 1.1). Everything here suggests maximum freedom and spontaneity, and it is tempting to imagine Beethoven at the keyboard playing this chord repeatedly until it reached what was for him the threshold of audibility. Where that threshold was reached is

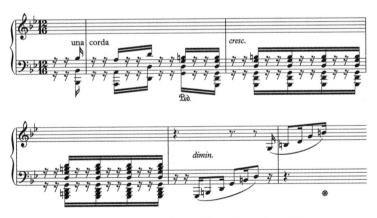

EXAMPLE 1.1. Beethoven, Piano Sonata in A-flat
Major, op. 110, 3rd movement, mm. 132–36

impossible to guess, since he did not specify the dynamic level at which the crescendo should peak. He himself was probably unsure, which is why the tenfold repetition was necessary. Perhaps he wrote it down in order to give posterity a glimpse into his workshop or to convey something of the uncertainty he felt in audible terms.

Let us likewise leave open the question of how complete Beethoven's deafness became during his final years. Terms like "stone deaf" and "completely unable to hear," which occur frequently in the Beethoven literature, are not particularly helpful, since the perception of sound is a complex phenomenon affected by many variables that may constantly be redefined. What is important to recognize is that Beethoven lived in an ongoing state of engagement with his disability. Once this is acknowledged, we can also understand how misleading it is to claim that he "overcame" his hearing loss. What he did was learn to work with and within it.

The same observation can be made about his personal life. When his first symptoms appeared, Beethoven feared that he would never again enjoy normal relations with other people, and his fears were justified. The difficult adjustments he had to make are usually viewed externally: Beethoven is seen as having become increasingly eccentric and difficult as he grew older. This was the perspective of people who knew and interacted with him. What the experience was like for Beethoven is, of course, much harder to imagine. Severe hearing loss is challenging enough today, when there are sophisticated hearing aids, closed captions, supportive communities, and a broad cultural sensitivity to the needs of people with disabilities. Beethoven had access to none of these things. The Austrian Taubstummeninstitut, or School for the Deaf and Dumb, had been founded in Vienna in 1779—one of the first institutions of its kind in Europe—and eventually became the center of a substantial deaf community.[59] There is no evidence, though, that Beethoven was aware of the existence of this community, let alone that he associated with it in any way. As we have seen, he consulted a long series of doctors, none of whom provided him with any help in dealing with his hearing loss. Therefore he was forced to confront it almost entirely alone. Helen Keller said that "blindness separates people from things; deafness separates people from people." Social isolation was not something that Beethoven chose, and his many eccentricities were not really free choices either; they were forced on him by circumstances and by the need to adapt.

It is hard to know how it felt to be in Beethoven's shoes. Nevertheless, there is a great deal to be learned from those who have followed in his footsteps.

* 2 *
2003: A Sudden Case of Deafness

Barbara was born in Pomona, at the foot of the San Gabriel Mountains and the entrance to Southern California's Inland Empire. In 1956 there were still orange groves and vineyards where now the imprint of Greater Los Angeles has blotted out local distinctions and absorbed former communities into its sameness: the sprawl of freeways, shopping malls, and housing tracts. Her parents were from opposite sides of the tracks in Chicago; her mother grew up in suburban, idyllic Glen Ellyn, while her father, the son of Austrian immigrants, lived in the gritty downtown around Damen Avenue. Born in 1925, he was rejected from service in World War II because he had contracted tuberculosis, and by the time he married his sweetheart in 1951 he had had a lung removed and was considered a poor prospect. Ironically, he was sent to California for the better air. He lived there until 2006, when he died of natural causes unrelated to the illness that had nearly killed him in his twenties.

Barbara was the third of four children born to Walter and Mary Lou Hutter. In 1961 they moved to the house in Ontario where her parents would live for nearly fifty years, the neighborhood and the canopy of trees slowly maturing around them. Ontario had been founded by a pair of Canadian brothers with a longing for their home province, and is now known primarily as the site of Greater Los Angeles's second largest airport. When I met Barbara in 1988 she was living in a condominium located on the flight path. As I drove in, it was not uncommon to see planes flying low enough to read the names of the airlines. Every ten minutes or so conversations would pause and TV volumes would be raised dramatically. There were still vineyards near the runway, although they were later removed when the airport was expanded to its present size.

Barbara attended the local public schools, graduating from Chaffey High School, a place that resembled a college campus, in 1974. Her father had begun teaching at what was then called Azusa Pacific College, where, after receiving his PhD from the Claremont Graduate School, he would later become dean of the School of Business. Barbara enrolled at AP and majored in nursing—her childhood ambition—receiving her BS and RN four years later, and began working med-surge at a local hospital. Then, in March 1979, as it had for her father at a similar age, her life took an inexplicable turn.

As March 16, her twenty-third birthday, approached, she began suffering from severe headaches. When they continued to grow worse, she went in for an emergency CT scan and received the grim news that she had a tumor in her right cerebellum. It had developed a cyst, which was causing the headaches and made emergency surgery an urgent necessity. The diagnosis was delivered on her birthday, and the surgery took place days later. Recently developed microsurgical techniques streamlined an operation that otherwise would have left her paralyzed. The tumor was removed, and a biopsy delivered the worst possible news: it was an astrocytoma, an aggressively malignant tumor that is almost always fatal. In the hopes of extending her life by a few years, radiation was administered repeatedly over the next few weeks. Nearly four decades ago, radiation treatment for cancer was still a blunt weapon; doses were large and targeting was crude. In order to reach her cerebellum effectively, the radiation had to be administered through her ears. Nobody thought about the long-term consequences, because the long term was then being measured in months, not years. Barbara's ears, though, were damaged to begin with. As a child she had suffered from repeated infections. Several times doctors lanced her eardrums: a painful procedure that may have relieved the infections but also cost her approximately 10 percent of her natural hearing. Although there were no tests immediately after her radiation, it was clear that it had damaged her hearing even further. Postsurgery she also experienced some problems with balance, persistent double vision, and nystagmus: an involuntary but persistent twitching of her eyes that made it even harder to concentrate visually. These problems were more bothersome than the hearing loss, so they received most of the clinical focus during her convalescence. Eventually the double vision subsided to something that emerged only when she was tired or under stress. The balance problems were brought under control. As for her hearing, it was adequate, so it was essentially ignored.

When I met Barbara in the spring of 1988, she had startled conventional wisdom by surviving for nine years with no further manifestations of cancer. Yearly MRIs had confirmed that the tumor site was essentially unchanged. The course of her life, though, had not been smooth. In 1983, less than four years after the cancer diagnosis, she had married Donald Sellers, a lieutenant in the United States Marine Corps. Barely over two years later he was killed, along with sixteen other marines, in a highly publicized helicopter crash near Okinawa. Barbara, who was pregnant with their child, miscarried a few weeks later.

It is hard to imagine how devastating these events must have been. Barbara's marriage to Don had been followed by the magical five-year "cancer free" pronouncement that finally allowed her to envision a future. The birth of a child would have been an investment in that future. Now, the marriage and the child both gone, she was once again adrift. It was only decades later, after her own death, that I fully understood the reserves of inner strength that she had to tap in order to become a survivor for the second time, still not out of her twenties. For three years she worked in a dermatologist's office, lived in the condo that she and Don had bought together, and, as she often put it, "just lived." When life loses its center, time moves forward but does not advance. The mourner marks time as others mark hours on a dull job or days in a long prison term; it passes unaccountably, without direction, the only relief offered by a weekend or a stint in the exercise yard, nothing to be envisioned or hoped beyond that small break in the routine. Barbara did well financially; life insurance and a military pension saw to that. She went on cruises, sang in choirs, visited Europe, maintained old friendships, dated sporadically, and visited regularly with her parents, who still lived a few miles away. It wasn't a bad life, but it was an empty one.

I met Barbara after spending the 1987–88 academic year at Scripps College in Claremont, the third temporary position I had obtained after receiving my PhD from Yale in 1984. Nowadays we would say that we met online. Back then it was called computer dating, and it seemed like a good option for a recently divorced man with no roots in the area. Being a "gypsy scholar" is easier than working as an adjunct—you at least receive benefits and a decent salary—but I had had to move cross-country three times in as many years, and one of the casualties was my marriage. Now I was at loose ends, having failed to secure a position for the next year despite glowing evaluations of my teaching and the publication of my first book to enthusiastic reviews. Only to another academic would this situation make sense. Barbara was baffled by it. But she was tired of drifting, and my sympathetic listening won her heart.

After I took her out for dinner for the first time, she temporarily lost her balance while getting into my car, which led to the story of the tumor and radiation. As we sat together in the parking lot on a California evening, she poured out her story, anger and frustration creeping out from behind her gentle demeanor. I took her hand and told of my own life: the brutal bullying throughout my years at school, the devastating depression that haunted my twenties, the ongoing frustration of a career unacknowledged by professional success. I assured her that God was not a sadist, even though we both felt a loathing for the seemingly manifest divine capriciousness that soured a faith neither of us was willing to abandon. As we talked, we were enveloped by a canopy of mutual understanding that remained a sacred space between the two of us through the twenty-four difficult years to come.

So we were married in January 1989, shortly after the lawsuit brought collectively by the widows of the marines killed in the crash was settled out of court. Each of the plaintiffs received a substantial monetary settlement. To this day I am grateful beyond words to Barbara for staking her future on me when I couldn't even get interviewed for a job—and this when a large sum of money was soon to come her way. We spent a week in Hawaii, living it up with a private plane tour of all the islands and dinner at Chez Paul, Maui's fabled five-star French restaurant. We got up before dawn to see the sun rise from atop Mauna Loa, and over mai tais and mahi mahi burgers we pondered the future. Barbara's life appeared far more secure than mine. She had a stable career. I was fully prepared to be a college professor, but it would take much anxious waiting, many compromises, and untold frustration to find a job. In the meantime I gave piano lessons, taught high school English, did private tutoring, and had the incomparable satisfaction of being a stay-at-home father after my daughter Jennifer was born. Ten years after receiving my PhD, I finally received my first offer of a tenure-track position, and, our family now completed by the arrival of our son Jeremy, we trekked across country to South Carolina, where I began teaching at Converse College in the fall. It felt like our lives had finally settled into place. For me it was the completion of a cycle. I had grown up in Oak Ridge, Tennessee, on the other side of the mountains. When I left for college I had been glad to get away from that part of the country. Now returning felt like going home.

By then, though, Barbara's hearing had grown considerably worse than it was when I first met her. This is not an easy thing to measure objectively. She had always had trouble participating in group conversations—a fact that she attributed to shyness but that probably had a hearing component as well. It is easier to concentrate on speaking to a single person than to deal with the interaction of many voices responding to and interrupting each other, punctuated by group laughter and other sounds. I suspect that Barbara often pretended to hear more than she did. Even in one-on-one exchanges she sometimes asked me to repeat myself, but of course everyone does that from time to time. It is hard to pinpoint when she began to do so more frequently.

One incident is particularly telling about the casual attitudes toward hearing loss that Barbara encountered. During one of the many follow-up visits to her surgery, she asked whether she should be concerned about her hearing. "Can you talk on the phone?" the doctor asked. "Yes," she said. "Then you're fine," he responded. Years later, she could still talk on the phone, and it didn't occur to her to question that doctor's snap judgment. What turned the tide was a community health fair in Ontario that we wandered into in 1992. Free hearing screenings were being offered, and Barbara decided to take one. She was told that she had significant hearing loss, particularly in her right ear, in which she had only about 60 percent of her normal hearing, and that she would benefit from a hearing aid. A few months later she got one, and she was wearing it when we moved across the country.

⁎

The resonances with Beethoven in this story are significant, despite the documentary vagueness that surrounds the onset of his hearing loss. Like Barbara's, Beethoven's began in his twenties, and while it may have had multiple causes, he and his contemporaries tended to trace it back to a single incident: a major illness or an accident. When I met Barbara she was thirty-two, a year older than Beethoven when he wrote the Heiligenstadt Testament. Like him, she had faced mounting symptoms for years but had tried to remain in denial about them. Barbara was not a trained musician, but she had always enjoyed singing in choirs—her mother was a church organist and choir director—and she continued to do so with no obvious difficulty even as her hearing deteriorated. She and I often attended concerts together, and her perception of live and recorded music did not appear to suffer. Only her understanding of speech was adversely affected, and it began to make her increasingly ill at ease socially.

Like Beethoven, Barbara experienced tinnitus more or less constantly after the radiation. This was something she got used to but also found barely tolerable at times. I quickly learned that "ringing in the ears" is not an adequate description of this curse. The sounds twisted and swelled in constant arabesques of shifting intensity. Sometimes they were high-pitched and shrill, while at other times they resembled the roar of a jet engine. They grew worse, or at least more noticeable, in the absence of other sounds, making the experience of silence a distant memory. They were often loudest when she was tired. I tried to understand that Barbara heard these sounds all the time; there was no way to make them stop. Earplugs were futile, since the sounds were coming from inside. The demon in her ears was a part of herself.

As these symptoms suggest, the hearing loss that Barbara experienced was primarily sensorineural. The radiation had damaged some of the hair cells in her cochlea, causing deficits that were particularly noticeable at certain pitches; there were a few unlucky people whom she could barely understand because they spoke almost entirely in a narrow range where she heard next to nothing. For the most part she was able to maintain the ruse of having normal hearing and being a bit socially awkward. In fact, until that hearing test at the health fair, that was what she firmly believed about herself. Again, the first symptoms of hearing loss are often subtle and easily explained away. It may be years before they are acknowledged for what they are.

That point was borne home in a stunning way a few years after our move to South Carolina. We made the three-hour drive to Knoxville to visit a friend of my mother's who specialized in helping people with hearing loss make use of what residual hearing they had left. He advised us that the hearing aid Barbara had been using was already outdated. At that point—the late 1990s—we faced a stark choice. High-tech hearing aids were available that cost over $20,000 and were so small as to be nearly undetectable. Or, for $1,000, we could buy an old-fashioned behind-the-ear hearing aid that would be glaringly obvious to everyone. Since hearing aids are not considered prosthetics and are hence not covered by insurance, the price difference was decisive. But the $1,000 aid was actually better; the huge cost of the smaller one served only to gratify the vanity of those who could afford it. Barbara, now in her early forties, had to decide that wearing an "I am hard of hearing" badge in public was preferable to sending the same message repeatedly in less obvious ways.

The day she tried out the new aid ranks as one of the most memorable in this entire story. Going for a walk outside the office, Barbara noticed the sound of a stream running nearby, "babbling" over rocks as streams do in many places in East Tennessee. She heard cars passing on the nearby street. With a shock of insight, she realized that she had not been hearing these things for a long time. Later, when we got in our car for the drive home, she began to expand the list of things she had not been hearing: the sounds of doors opening; the click-click of the turn signal; the explosion of ice into the cup as we stopped for a fountain drink at a local convenience store. She was suddenly overwhelmed with sound, and it was at first a bit disconcerting. I could understand this because I had had a similar experience several times after having a large buildup of wax removed from my ears. Afterward, the field of auditory information I was receiving expanded dramatically. Footsteps were small thuds; putting the key in the lock of the car door was a symphony of metal scraping on internal parts and shifting them into place. These are things we hear all the time and barely notice because we take them for granted. The realization that you have not been hearing them, though, brings them forth in their full sonic complexity. You are suddenly surrounded by an unfathomable abundance of sound, which overwhelms you until you learn again to turn it into a gentle backdrop for the more important sounds that you actually need to hear: the shout, the siren, the voices of those near you. That day, Barbara had that experience on a scale of magnitude I had never imagined.

The long-term benefits were much less dramatic. Her speech comprehension improved, but she still had trouble in large groups or noisy public situations. Eventually she got a hearing aid for her left ear too, but the benefits of this one were even more subtle: less head-turning when people spoke to her from the wrong side, perhaps a bit more accuracy in directional perception. Her experience of music did not appear to change; throughout the long decline of her hearing she sang in the alto section of our church choir and had no trouble matching pitches and blending with the other singers.

The first sign of more serious problems with Barbara's health came in March 2000, just days after her forty-fourth birthday. I was away for the weekend at a regional academic conference in Greensboro, NC, that I had helped organize. On the drive home I stopped and called Barbara—this was before we had cell phones—and learned that she had been seeing flashing lights for several hours. This was apparently an ocular migraine, of the kind that she had experienced her entire adult life, but a particularly vehement one.

It has been suggested that the visions of the medieval abbess Hildegard von Bingen were similar migraine "auras." Of one such vision, Hildegard wrote: "I saw a great star most splendid and beautiful, and with it an exceeding multitude of falling stars which with the star followed southwards. . . . And suddenly they were all annihilated, being turned into black coals . . . and cast into the abyss so that I could see them no more."[1] This description is quoted in a book on migraine by Oliver Sacks, who goes on to explain the phenomenon more prosaically: "Our literal interpretation would be that she experienced a shower of phosphenes in transit across the visual field, their passage being succeeded by a negative scotoma."[2] Barbara called these events her "sparklies," and they normally occurred once or twice a month, usually in only one eye but sometimes in both. The lights would flash and sparkle with growing intensity for about twenty minutes, after which they would begin to fade. This one showed no sign of abating, and when it was still going on two days later I took her to the hospital, where a CT scan showed nothing unusual going on.

The next morning the flashing was growing worse, and Barbara was scared out of her wits. We waylaid our neighbor, a physician, before he left for work, and he performed a few quick tests and sent her back to the emergency room. That night, as I was grading assignments from one of my classes, another doctor told Barbara she was having a stroke and admitted her overnight. By this time the right side of her field of vision was almost entirely gone, and for nearly two months afterward she could see only things on her left until normal vision gradually returned. She was physically weak and highly emotional: both typical of patients who have suffered strokes. The official diagnosis was "migraine-induced stroke," or, as another doctor later put it, "a really nasty migraine." (None of these events, incidentally, ever involved a headache.) The location of the stroke was in her cerebellum, near where the tumor had been.

Then, in July of the same year, she woke up one morning and couldn't hear anything out of her right ear. Getting out of bed she fell flat on her face, unable to maintain her balance, and had to crawl to the bathroom. It was clear that something significant had happened in her inner or middle ear, where balance as well as hearing is centered. This single incident was far more dramatic than anything that happened to Beethoven, unless we accept the story of him falling to the floor in 1796; all but about 3 percent of the hearing in Barbara's right ear was now gone, never to return, and she would be vexed by severe balance problems for the remainder of her life. Yet, despite consultations with several local doctors and multiple trips to the Duke Medical Center—a four-hour drive away—for further testing, it was not until December that we received a definitive diagnosis. Modern medicine was baffled by this event: a fact that puts the multiple diagnoses and confusion surrounding Beethoven's hearing loss two hundred years earlier into perspective. Hearing loss is still not easy to explain.

The first diagnosis we received was dropsy: the middle ear had become filled with fluid, which was blocking sound from entering. Barbara was prescribed an extensive course of diuretics to drain the liquid. Day after day we waited for an indication that her hearing was starting to return. Day after day there was no change, and over the next few months it began to appear much more likely that the hearing in her right ear was gone for good.

Sudden hearing loss stories began to pour in; I was startled and a bit alarmed to learn how many people seemed to know someone who one day woke up deaf, usually for reasons that weren't immediately clear. Anecdotally, it seemed that this could result from a virus, from circulatory events, or from several other obscure causes. Nobody's hearing appeared to be safe.

Meanwhile, Barbara also had to deal with the loss of her balance. After that first morning she learned that she could walk on both feet, but it required considerable effort and she appeared to stagger like a drunk. Only gradually did this improve, and by the fall she still often needed to take my arm in public in order to stay upright. She would never walk with full confidence again.

It soon became evident that Barbara could no longer work as a registered nurse. Since I began teaching at Converse, she had held a series of part-time jobs, mostly in home health care. She visited patients who had been released from the hospital but still needed wounds dressed, vitals taken, and other routine tasks performed. We had arranged our schedules so she did this mainly in the late afternoon, in early evening, and on weekends so that someone was always home with our children. Having her work these hours was a financial necessity; as an assistant professor I wasn't paid enough for a family of four to live on. Now Barbara found that with only one ear—and that one compromised—she couldn't hear well enough with a stethoscope to take blood pressures. This plus her trouble walking upright made work nearly impossible. We decided to withdraw some of the remaining money from her financial settlement over Don's death, which had been sitting in a mutual fund intended to cover college costs for our children, and after twenty-two years Barbara's career as a nurse was over.

This was also the point that music began to be a problem for her. With only one working ear, she found that she could no longer hear the other singers in the choir well enough to blend in. She had been singing in choirs since high school—much longer than she had been a nurse—and now with great regret she had to give that up as well. She could still enjoy listening, but for the first time she began saying that the sounds she heard were significantly distorted, particularly at live performances, and her pleasure in music decreased. We attended a concert by Peter Schickele, known as the "discoverer" of P. D. Q. Bach. Much of his work depends on amusing audiences by producing unusual instrumental sounds. Barbara found this deeply confusing; much of the time she was not sure whether she was hearing what she was supposed to be hearing and whether she should laugh or not.

Listening to live speech also became more challenging. Previously Barbara had had no major trouble following lectures or going to the theater or movies, despite her difficulties with group conversations. Now she found it necessary to sit in the very front rows, much as Beethoven did at the time of his letter to Wegeler. We found that this could have its advantages. Our daughter Jennifer was dancing in a production of *The Nutcracker*, and relatives were coming from out of town. The production was nearly sold out, and I was hoping that explaining Barbara's handicap would help us get better seats. As soon as I said that my wife was deaf in one ear, I was told that the entire first two rows of the theater were blocked out for people with audiovisual handicaps and their companions. All of us enjoyed the close-up view, and Barbara, of course, heard much better than she would have if we had sat farther back.

✳

Meanwhile, the quest for a diagnosis continued. Our final trip to the Duke Medical Center took place in the midst of the Supreme Court case over the contested 2000 presidential election, which played out on television screens everywhere we stopped along the way like an ironic backdrop to our personal uncertainty. On an earlier visit Barbara had undergone rotational testing, which involved being spun around in a chair, and some advanced visioning procedures to get a closer look at her middle and inner ears. The results were in, and they showed that she had had another stroke: a spasm in the internal auditory artery, which supplies blood to the cochlea and the vestibular system.[3] This had cut off the supply of oxygen long enough that nearly all of the hair cells in the cochlea had died. Since those cells supply the information that the brain translates into sound, their loss en masse meant deafness. There were only two ways that the lost hearing might be recovered; one of them sounded like science fiction, and the other would have sounded like science fiction if it were not already real.

The sci-fi option was hair cell regeneration. Each ear contains around twenty thousand hair cells, which play a key role in transforming vibrations entering the ear into neural information that the brain registers as sound. These are the crux of the sense of hearing; if they die, they cannot be replaced, and the result is sensorineural deafness. Human hair cells are incapable of regeneration, so such deafness is considered permanent. Already in 2000 researchers were talking about overcoming this challenge, and we were encouraged to hope that their efforts would bear fruit during our lifetimes.

The non-sci-fi option was the cochlear implant. Since the 1970s doctors had been implanting minicomputers into people's heads and connecting them via electrodes to the cochlea and hence to the auditory nerve so they could relay electric signals that would register as sound. By 2000 these devices were advanced enough to operate with sixteen different channels, and were sufficiently mainstream to be covered by medical insurance. Barbara was not eligible, though, because she still had a "good" ear, and insurance would not cover an implant—at a cost of close to $100,000—for a patient who was not deaf in both. Furthermore, getting an implant would destroy the cochlea, ruling out hair cell regeneration in the future. So cochlear implantation was put on hold, and we were sent home with a diagnosis but no treatment. There was also an ominous takeaway: All of the blood vessels in Barbara's head had been damaged by the radiation, making them about fifteen years older than her physical age. At forty-four, she had the brain circulation of a woman nearing sixty, and perhaps even older. The vulnerability to stroke that had been established by the past year's events did not bode well for the future. The doctor advised her to exercise every day and take extra care of her circulatory health to safeguard the hearing in her remaining ear.

☀

In the fall of 2001, on the advice of the local disability office, Barbara began retraining for a career as a medical insurance specialist. This would allow her to work in an office, remain in the medical field, and put her knowledge to use without great demands on her mobility or hearing. It required taking classes for two years at the local technical college. This proved to be the greatest challenge yet, because hearing the professor, let alone the comments and questions of the other students, was often beyond her. Eventually the college provided her with an FM system that broadcast the professor's voice directly into a set of headphones that she wore. It still wasn't easy, and there were days when she was so frustrated with her situation she was near despair. She persisted, though, until finally toward the end of her training she began to work with insurance codes.

This was when she realized that the stroke in March 2000 had left her with a lingering visual aphasia, even though her eyesight seemed to have returned to normal. She would look at a string of numbers and not see one of them. She didn't see a blank or a blur; she simply saw the other numbers as one continuous sequence from which nothing appeared to be missing. Later this aphasia would manifest in other ways as well. She would be reading something and realize it didn't make sense; going back over it, she would notice there was a word she hadn't seen the first time through. She would be looking for something in the kitchen and not be able to see it until it was pointed out to her. Problems like this were frustrating, but they could be dealt with. Medical insurance filing, though, requires absolutely accurate transcription of countless numerical codes; a single error can cause a claim to be rejected. But Barbara didn't know when she was missing something, because the codes didn't need to make sense. It was literally impossible for her to be confident that her work was accurate, and proofreading was useless. She was manifestly unqualified for the job she had just spent two years retraining to do.

In the ongoing saga of Barbara's hearing loss and attempts to accommodate it, this would have been a low point of unimaginable pathos but for the fact that it was immediately followed by the loss of the hearing in her remaining ear. As it was, two gates were slammed shut with stereophonic precision in early 2003.

It had been a more severe winter than usual in upstate South Carolina. Because of an ice storm just before Christmas, we lost our power for nearly a week and had to abandon our unheated house for a hotel room. During this time I received a letter inviting me to apply for a job at Baylor University, and the idea of a move seemed suddenly enticing. The process of applying for an academic job is a long and involved one that I had initiated countless times during my years of underemployment. For nine years I had relished not having to think about doing it again. This time I applied only to this one position. A few months later I was invited to campus for an interview.

The weather in Waco, Texas, in early March was California perfect. My interactions with students, faculty, and administration were positive and encouraging. As the semester at Converse drew to an end and the reality sank in that Barbara had spent two years retraining for a job she would never be able to do, I was offered the position at Baylor with tenure and 65 percent higher pay than I was receiving. Some believe in serendipity, others in divine providence. In Shakespeare's words, "There is a tide in the affairs of men, which taken at the flood leads on to fortune." We had had enough of shallows and miseries, and Barbara and I seized the tide, hoping at least to remain afloat and at best to prosper.

It was on the morning in June that we were preparing to drive to Waco and pick out a house that Barbara suddenly lost the hearing in her remaining ear. This time it didn't happen in her sleep. She was lifting a box when she heard a *pfwit!* noise and was then unable to hear anything. As it turned out, not even 3 percent of her left-ear hearing remained as it did in the right ear. In less than a second, all remaining hearing in her left ear simply vanished.

Because I was pretty sure I knew what was happening this time, I rushed Barbara to the hospital. In the introduction to this book I described the sheer devastation caused by the onset of total deafness. The mix of emotions I felt as I waited for news in the emergency room while placing calls to family members was more complex. I am ashamed to admit I felt anger: anger at being once again in this place fraught with memories of past crises; anger at Barbara for having practically ignored the doctor's advice to get regular exercise if she didn't want to lose what was left of her hearing. I had tried to find gentle but persistent ways to remind her of this, and had largely failed. Now I couldn't shake my sense of grievance that if she had only listened, I would not be pacing these floors again. I also hoped against hope that if the blockage of the blood flow to her inner ear could be stopped or lessened in time, at least some of her hair cells could recover. It was hard to believe that oxygen deprivation had killed them all in such a short time. The ER doctor's decision to inject cortisone was encouraging, as was his suggestion that the hearing could start to come back any time over the next week or two if we continued the procedure. We were supposed to have gone to Knoxville that day and left the children with my mother while we drove on to Texas. We ended up meeting her and her husband for dinner at a Cracker Barrel west of Asheville before they took Jennifer and Jeremy home for a week so Barbara and I could take stock of our lives.

I don't think I really believed her hearing would come back. For the next two weeks we trudged dutifully to a specialist's office to have the painful cortisone injections repeated. We were told that if any change was going to come it would happen gradually. We anxiously waited for some sign that she might be starting to hear even a whisper of the surrounding world, until at last it was painfully obvious that such hope was a chimera. "I'm sorry," the doctor finally said, and with those words closed off one avenue of hope even as his next words opened another: "A cochlear implant is in your future."

So we drove to Texas suspended between one life and another, unable to have a two-way conversation that was not half written down. One particularly poignant moment stands out: On the first day, having stopped for dinner, we went to a pay phone at a mall to call and check in with the kids, who were staying at our home with Barbara's parents. Barbara could only stand and watch while I did the talking. A mother completely cut off from her children: I watched her diminish in her own eyes as the weight of this reality settled upon her. Then we got back into the car and drove off into the gathering dusk.

⁎

The next few months were like Beethoven's experience condensed into a shorter and more challenging time frame. Like Beethoven, Barbara found herself isolated socially to a degree that had not seemed possible before the catastrophe set in. Absolutely everything that was said to her had to be written down. No interaction with groups was possible. She couldn't hear what was said at church, which had always been an anchor for her life. Public entertainment was off limits. Music vanished. The world became a prison cell devoid of anything beyond its gray concrete walls.

Barbara did have a few communication options that were not open to Beethoven, and these were a lifeline. She could at least watch TV, since by this time all programming was closed captioned. She could access the internet and converse with people by instant message. Taking a break from the cumbersome conversation books, I sometimes "talked" with her at the computer; she stood or sat beside me and spoke while I typed my responses.

What both of us noticed about that time was the grieving, which we shared even though Barbara bore the heavier burden. What had happened felt like a death, and we began recognizing it as such almost immediately. It was the death of much of our previous married life, of many of our shared dreams, of our ability to listen to music together or to enjoy spontaneous family time unburdened by the struggle to communicate. We both mourned, and in the process dark and powerful emotions surged through us that hurt us deeply yet paradoxically offered relief. We learned to face death together, and this earlier death began to prepare me for Barbara's actual death eight and a half years later. The emotions we shared continued to resonate through my life and sustained me after she was no longer physically present. Like a grand and tragic piece of music, Barbara's sudden and devastating loss echoed forward in time and in turn inspired others who witnessed our response to it.

We moved to Texas at the beginning of August, and the social isolation became much worse. Barbara knew nobody in Waco and had no way of making contacts. The Deaf community was off limits because she did not sign. We began to visit the cochlear implant community in Dallas, but here too she did not fit in since she could still hear nothing. We began attending a new church, which used liturgies we had never heard before. As longtime Lutherans, though, we easily fell into the rhythm of the service: the printed prayers and responses, the familiar sections whose words we knew by heart, the unfolding rhythm of the liturgy that led, cadence by cadence, to the peroration of Communion, blessing, and dismissal. "Thanks be to God," we responded at the end, and meant it. Without being able to hear a single note or a single word, Barbara was caught up in the music she knew so well.

With Barbara's implantation later that fall began a new stage of the journey: one in which she would not regain normal hearing but would learn, as far as possible, to live and work within the new limits set by her disability. Here her experience and that of Beethoven harmonize again, but it will take the next two chapters just to begin teasing out the subtle and complex counterpoint that links them together.

* 3 *
The Deaf Composer

Ludwig van Beethoven was many things: a pianist, a celebrated improviser, a conductor, an erratic and larger-than-life personality who charmed and frightened people by turns. He is remembered today, though, for being a composer. He wrote music—great music that resounds in concert halls throughout the world nearly two hundred years after his death.

But what does it mean to write music? How did Beethoven become known above all for his written works? The answer is complex—far more complex than the simple fact that he continued composing after his growing deafness cut short his career as a performer.

Most music is never written down. This fact seems obvious to popular musicians and to those from non-European cultures, but the history of Western classical music is often told in a way that obscures and even ignores it. Though we know that Bach, Mozart, and Beethoven were all celebrated for their improvisations, when we study their music, we study written scores. Performers who are faithful to what the composer wrote often receive more respect than those who take liberties with it. Few musicians trained in the Western classical repertory learn to improvise, and even fewer to improvise well.

Most students are taught to read music as soon as they begin to play.

In the eighteenth century things were different. As Robert Gjerdingen has pointed out, like other beginning students of the time Mozart learned to "speak" music before he learned to read it.[1] His earliest compositions were written down by his father, who continued to assist him for several years. Like a child learning a language, Mozart developed his verbal and aural skills first. When he performed publicly throughout Europe as a child, he improvised, sometimes blindfolded. Later in life he did the same thing minus the blindfold, much to the enjoyment of his audiences, who did not want or expect to hear something they had heard before.

We know much less about Beethoven's early training than we do about Mozart's, but we can probably assume it followed a similar pattern. European music in the mid-eighteenth century was an elaborate language that sprang from Italian soil and was often called by the French name *galant*.[2] Understanding this term is a key to understanding Beethoven, who like others of his time grew up with *galant* as his native musical language, but later wrote music that those accustomed to the *galant* style found challenging or even incomprehensible. Something of what it meant to be *galant* can be garnered from the writings of Bernard le Bovier de Fontenelle (1657–1757), whose *Conversations on the Plurality of Worlds* went through many editions and became one of the most widely read books of its time. Well aware of the fates of Giordano Bruno and Galileo, who were persecuted for their then-outlandish scientific ideas, Fontenelle couched his speculations about the solar system and life on other planets in the form of a series of witty and flirtatious dialogues between a narrator and a beautiful, clever noblewoman. Although Fontenelle was well grounded in the most advanced scientific knowledge of his time, the book can be read purely for entertainment and its imaginative descriptions of other worlds taken as whimsy rather than as challenges to received wisdom. The *galant* knew how to be sophisticated and self-deprecating at the same time, how to say a lot without violating the codes of polite society. *Galant* music strove for the same goal.

Gjerdingen has shown that the standard vocabulary of mid-eighteenth-century music was shaped not just by melodic patterns and harmonic sequences but by standard schemata in which the two were combined in characteristic ways. The schemata were themselves joined in broadly understood patterns that could be manipulated with the same virtuosic flexibility found in the improvised theater style known as commedia dell'arte, in which actors practiced standard speeches, exchanges, and comedic tricks until they could string them together in various ways so their performances seemed continually fresh.[3] This was the art of improvisation, and musicians of the time learned to do the same thing. Like jazz musicians of today, though perhaps to a lesser degree, performers understood the written score as a starting point, not an inviolable set of instructions.

Written compositions were themselves a kind of improvisation on paper. Composers, like performers, would combine conventional musical gestures and patterns in novel—and often not particularly novel—ways. Because the underlying musical language and its conventions were so broadly shared, eighteenth-century composers like Georg Philip Telemann—the author of more than three thousand works—were able to write music in mind-boggling quantities.

Beyond the *Galant*

Beethoven famously accomplished two seemingly contradictory things: composing laboriously and improvising brilliantly. He devoted more time and paper to the act of composing each of his works than perhaps anyone who came before him. As a result, he wrote a relatively small number of pieces by eighteenth-century standards—9 symphonies to Haydn's 104, for example. He also improvised with confidence and panache, producing music on the spot that thrilled and amazed his listeners. The skill set required to do one of these things would appear to be the opposite of that needed to do the other. This seeming enigma can be resolved if we understand that all competent musicians in Beethoven's time knew how to improvise and did so more or less constantly within well-established frameworks. On the other hand, when musicians like Mozart and C. P. E. Bach published works titled *Fantasy, Fantasia, Phantasie,* or *Fantaisie*—the word signified free improvisation in virtually all European languages—these pieces were usually full of stark contrasts, sudden transitions, and novel effects. In order to sound like you were improvising, you were expected to keep your audience on the edge of their seats, bombarding them with unexpected tricks and seemingly new ideas. This strategy was so well understood that a published piece titled *Capriccio, Fantasy,* or *Impromptu* could be received without irony.

Early reviews of Beethoven show that even his works that were not so titled often struck his first hearers as improvisations or fantasies, leaving them confused and disoriented. Reading between the lines, we understand that composers carefully cultivated the improvisational manner to impress listeners with its seeming spontaneity, but such spontaneity was not always welcome in a work claiming to be a sonata or a symphony.[4] Beethoven's public improvisations were impressive precisely because he had worked so hard behind the scenes at producing effects that seemed to emerge without premeditation. When he did the same thing in print, he was castigated for it instead of being applauded.

What Beethoven's improvisations and his published works had in common was that they defied the *galant* ideal of light, gracious, civilized discourse. That ideal was itself a product of severe and self-conscious discipline, so Beethoven's transformation of it could easily seem impulsive and arbitrary. It was in fact the exact opposite: his was a deliberate act of composition that changed the received vocabulary of music. Beethoven produced works that often went beyond established formulas and conventions, or retained them only to adapt them to deeply personal aims. What these works lost in universal accessibility they gained in depth of expression and variety.

For Beethoven, composing music meant walking through the streets of Vienna and the surrounding countryside, music paper in hand. It involved stormy sessions at the piano in which he worked out his ideas, and others at his desk when he sketched at lightning speed or filled his manuscripts with last-minute corrections. He used the piano to the limit of its capabilities and used paper in profligate abundance. He fully exploited every physical medium available to him. For Beethoven music was always more than sound. It was a map of his inner experience, expressed outwardly through extravagant gestures, virtuosic use of the keyboard, and constant, compulsive writing and revising. Deafness was not about to derail him.

How Did He Do It?

When people learn that Beethoven composed music despite being deaf, the most commonly asked question is, How did he do it? Like flying without wings, composing without hearing seems like a violation of physics: a quixotic attempt to travel through a medium that will not support one's weight. But the medium through which Beethoven and other composers travel is richly multifaceted. Music originates in the body, and composers often work with an instrument, with paper, and with a pen or pencil. Even before his deafness began Beethoven was using all of these in novel ways. Later he would add ear trumpets and a resonator to the mix, would stuff his ears with cotton, and would devote perhaps more time than ever to the writing process. He would increasingly retreat from performing and would demand louder instruments for himself to play. Fundamentally, though, what he did remained the same. He improvised at the piano. He sketched. He revised. He drew music from the intersection of his physical presence with the materials of his craft. It would be misleading to say that he did these things in exactly the same way after he became unable to hear. But it would be equally misleading to suggest that he simply "heard the music in his head" and wrote it down.

There is a well-known scene in *Amadeus* in which Mozart, on his deathbed, dictates the "Confutatis" from the *Requiem* to his fellow composer Antonio Salieri, one part at a time. Salieri painstakingly takes down the notes, and then the movie's musical score dramatically shifts to a performance of the fully orchestrated piece, sounding just as we are encouraged to believe that Mozart heard it in his imagination.

This depiction of Mozart's creative process is based on a well-known letter that first appeared in the highly influential journal *Allgemeine musikalische Zeitung* in 1815. Writing to an unspecified baron, Mozart supposedly said this about his method of composing:

> I can really say nothing more about it than this, since I know nothing more about it myself and cannot explain it further. Ideas are most likely to rush upon me when I am entirely alone and in good spirits, perhaps traveling in a carriage, or taking a walk after a good meal, or at night when I can't sleep. I don't know where they come from or how, and I can't coerce them. I retain those I like in my head, and, as

others have confirmed, I hum them to myself. If I preserve one of these crumbs, I quickly see how it can be made progressively into a pastry through counterpoint, through the sounds of various instruments, etc., etc., etc. This excites my soul, and if I am not disturbed it becomes ever greater, and I expand it ever more broadly and clearly, and the thing is practically finished in my head, be it ever so long, so that henceforth I can take it in at a single glance, like a pretty picture or an attractive person.[5]

By the time he wrote a piece down, Mozart is supposed to have claimed, it was already finished in all its essential details.

Scholars have long known that this familiar account, widely cited by later writers, is a transparent forgery. It suited nineteenth-century ideas about creativity to suggest that a complete work could take shape in a composer's mind without the use of an instrument or paper, but Mozart never claimed to have worked in this way. Neither did Beethoven, although a close paraphrase of the spurious Mozart letter was ascribed to him by his biographer Louis Schlösser and appeared in English in O. G. Sonneck's influential *Beethoven: Impressions by His Contemporaries*.[6] Generations of readers have thus grown up with a mistaken impression of how both composers worked.

At the Piano

The reality was far more complex, and far more interesting. Since Beethoven was a pianist, his musical ideas reflected his experience with that instrument. Here he stood at a watershed. Pianos had existed since 1700, when the first one was manufactured by Bartolomeo Cristofori in Florence.[7] For most of the eighteenth century, though, the piano was the least popular keyboard instrument, second to the harpsichord and the clavichord; it hit its stride only in the 1780s and 90s. Growing up in Bonn, Beethoven probably received much of his early training on a clavichord, a small and simple instrument with a very quiet tone but capable of great expressive nuance.[8] Only in his mid- to late teens did he become broadly familiar with the piano, and he quickly developed an idiosyncratic playing style, which included a preference for producing a "singing" tone at that instrument as well.[9]

The idea that a piano can sing is counterintuitive. It is a percussion instrument; the notes, produced by a hammer striking the strings, have a sharp onset and decay quickly. By contrast, singers—at least in the Western classical tradition—sustain notes and join them together to produce smooth, flowing phrases. Along with others of his generation, Beethoven had the challenge of figuring out how to imitate this at the piano. To learn how to do so, he would have had to experiment tenaciously. Even today, when the idea that a piano should sing is widely accepted, there is no formula for producing this kind of tone. It requires full sensory and physical engagement; the player must listen carefully and modify his or her technique, then continue to participate in an ongoing feedback loop between ears and fingers. Beethoven had practically no previous examples to go on, so he faced the challenge of producing what he came to call "my own tone" by himself.[10] Eventually, after an untold amount of private practice, frustration, and sweat, he learned to make the piano sing with a degree of automaticity, while also perfecting other aspects of his distinctive sound. Like all good performers, he was no longer conscious of the individual steps by which he produced his characteristic sound. The tones that emerged from his instrument became extensions of himself.

As Beethoven lost his hearing, his ability to play with a singing tone would have been compromised. Other aspects of piano playing, though, might have had greater staying power. Pianists learn how to play scales and arpeggios, how to shape the hand around chords, how to produce sonorities both massive and thin by adding and subtracting notes and force. They learn how it feels to slip from one key into another or to enrich a familiar harmony with extra notes. Eventually, as with tone production, their fingers begin to do these things automatically. Beethoven could never have achieved fame as an improviser if his hands had not acquired a mind of their own, acting in advance of any feedback from his ears. Reports indicate that Beethoven could improvise effectively even at the very end of his life, long after he had ceased to play in public.[11] We may assume that, like his manner of tone production, such improvisation arose from his entire body and hence was not constrained by what he was able to hear. After his deafness became impossible to deny, he grew increasingly dissatisfied with the limits of the pianos at his disposal, whereas earlier he seems to have been willing to work within those limits.[12] He also gave increasing attention to the physical act of writing music, gradually working out a new and far-reaching relationship with what in German are called *die Noten*: the notes. More than any previous composer, Beethoven used notation to shape sound, letting his eyes take the lead where his ears could no longer easily follow.

Pen and Paper

Sketches by Beethoven survive from his years in Bonn, but after he moved to Vienna he devoted more and more attention to formulating his thoughts on paper, with results that have intrigued scholars and sometimes puzzled them. Commenting on a sketch sheet from the mid-1790s, Joseph Kerman pointed out:

These sketches are really very strange. The work they re-cord is work that anyone else would have done at the pi-ano, not at the writing desk. Yet even at the height of his fame as a pianist, when deafness was an as yet unsuspected nightmare, Beethoven seems to have experienced a com-pulsion to get things down on paper—not only musical autographs but also drafts of all kinds, sketches of all kinds, notions, memoranda, and the most picayune of composi-tional tinkerings. He had a veritable commitment to the graphic act.[13]

Even in his finished manuscripts there is often evidence that writing for Beethoven was a kind of performance. "Beethoven not only recorded but experienced his music as he wrote it down," writes William Newman. "Thus, often when his phrases and subphrases swell and diminish, his notation slants forward and straightens up again, as on the opening page of the 'Appas-sionata' Sonata Op. 57. When the tempo presses forward, so does the notation . . . when the tempo holds back, again so does the notation. . . . When the staccatos grow crisper and brighter, the dots tend to change gradually to strokes."[14]

As with improvisation and tone production at the piano, Beethoven's writing process was personal and central to his identity. The satisfaction he got from this process could not have been purely intellectual. He was not merely writing down ideas; he was generating them. In Schlösser's forged recollec-tion, Beethoven supposedly said: "I carry my thoughts about with me for a long time, sometimes a very long time, before I set them down."[15] In fact he carried his sketches with him for a very long time and rarely went anywhere without paper on which to write. According to Schlösser, "The working out in breadth, length, height and depth begins in my head, and since I am conscious of what I want, the basic idea never leaves me."[16] Instead that working out began on paper or at the keyboard, and the fear that the basic idea might leave him seems to have driven him to extraordinary efforts to refine and perfect it in writing.

What these examples suggest is that the way Beethoven composed music was determined by habits that were particular to him and that were established early in his life. As his hearing deteriorated his working method developed further, but it did so on a continuum; there was no dramatic change, no before deafness and after deafness. There was only an ongoing refinement of his relationship with the piano—which itself was undergoing constant changes in structure and design—and of the way he worked on paper as his hearing deteriorated.

It is even possible that there is a simple explanation for the "strangeness" of some of Beethoven's early sketches. After Barbara lost her hearing, she found that she had already acquired considerable skill in lipreading without realizing it. Over the years—beginning perhaps before I knew her—she had begun to use her eyes to fill in gaps in what she heard people say, even though she did not yet believe her hearing needed help. She grew in the habit of turning her head toward the person who was speaking, and it was only after the remainder of her hearing suddenly disappeared that she understood how much she had been using the information she received this way to fill in for phonemes that her ears did not quite register. She then began to consciously augment the skill she had already acquired.[17]

It seems more than likely that Beethoven's sketches from his early twenties show a similar mix of self-awareness and lack of it. While deafness may have been "an as yet unsuspected nightmare," it is possible, as noted in chapter 1, that Beethoven's hearing began to fail long before he admitted it even to himself. If asked to explain his devotion to the writing process at this early point in his career, he might not have acknowledged that it helped his musical imagination construct things he was not quite able to arrive at using his ears alone—or if he did acknowledge it, he might not have admitted that he needed paper to make up for a deficit in his hearing. Only after his deafness grew worse did he realize how important the written page had become to him. Like Barbara, who belatedly realized that lipreading helped her to understand speech and then applied herself to learning to do it better, Beethoven, as he approached thirty, dedicated himself to sketching and revising with renewed vigor, gathering sketch leaves together and binding them into the sketchbooks that he would use for the rest of his life.

The creation of the first sketchbooks in 1798 can be attributed solely to the fact that Beethoven needed to give painstaking focus to his work on Opus 18, his first set of string quartets and hence the first work in which he engaged directly with the legacy of Mozart and Haydn.[18] But he might also have decided to accept the challenge of writing those quartets, which he had declined earlier, because his creative intuition—his daimon, to use a more venerable term—told him it was a good idea to refine and expand his technique on paper while he could still hear. In either case the result was the same: as he heard less, he wrote more, and once established, that correlation continued for the rest of his life. Nevertheless, he continued to work at the keyboard as well; the year before he died he still kept a table covered with sketches next to his piano so he could write down ideas as he improvised them.[19] The way he composed music had not fundamentally changed.

So the best answer to the question "How did he do it?" is "The same way he always did." Rather than envisioning the deaf Beethoven as a bird without wings or a fish out of water, we might think of him as a pilot flying safely without working navigational instruments, but with a deep bodily knowledge of how to steer an aircraft. The analogy is imperfect, of course. A plane can crash, whereas a deaf composer can do no worse than write music that people dislike.

Late Beethoven

In fact, immediately after Beethoven's death, two major articles appeared, read by musicians throughout the German-speaking world, suggesting that this was exactly what had happened. Beethoven's later works were insane, incomprehensible, because he was no longer writing "music for the ears."[20] In the words of the Berlin critic Ernst Woldemar, Beethoven

> did not pay the slightest attention, in his last compositions, to the Horatian canon: "*sit, quodvis, simplex duntaxat et unum*" (whatever you undertake to create, let it at least be simple and a whole), which applies to all the fine arts. He writes far out into the blue (with, to be sure, a level of imagination that is still gigantic, but is only to the worse without the firm hand of self-possessed criticism!), untroubled by how things turn out.

Woldemar wrote that on hearing Beethoven's late works, he felt like he was "in nothing other than a madhouse, and . . . must accordingly find them to be in fact most horrible, tasteless, and dreadful."[21]

Similar opinions were frequently stated in the decades that followed, even by highly sympathetic listeners.[22] As a result, a complex mythology has arisen concerning Beethoven's "late" style, the last of his three major style periods, which is usually seen as beginning with the Piano Sonata in A Major, op. 101, and the two cello sonatas of Opus 102. That style is also understood to include the four piano sonatas that followed, the last five string quartets, the Ninth Symphony, the *Missa Solemnis*, the Diabelli variations, and some minor works like the last two sets of bagatelles for piano, opp. 119 and 126. Compared to the works of the early period (up to 1803) and the middle period (1803–ca. 1814), the works of the late period are usually heard today as more personal, more intimate, and also more difficult to understand. From the very first, though, these pieces were understood as products of Beethoven's deafness. For many of their first hearers, this meant they were defective.

For others, the fact that this music was written when Beethoven was deaf was a proof of its greatness. K. M. Knittel has suggested that it was Wagner's romanticizing of deafness, which he came to see as an idyllic escape from the noise and conflict of the modern world, that allowed later critics to reevaluate Beethoven's late music in a more sympathetic light.[23] The reevaluation, though, had started much earlier—virtually as soon as the late works appeared. In the words of Nicholas Cook: "If it had been an unheard-of young composer who presented the Viennese public of the 1820s with the Ninth Symphony or the 'Hammerklavier' Sonata, they would almost certainly have been dismissed as bizarre and incompetent." Cook's statement may seem baffling to modern readers, for many of whom Beethoven's Ninth Symphony is the virtual epitome of classical music, but at first hearing, this work, like the *Hammerklavier*, op. 106, presented unprecedented challenges by virtue of its enormous length and highly idiosyncratic style. By the time these works appeared, though, Cook suggests, "the musical public had a massive emotional investment in [Beethoven's] music. . . . And so his many devotees set themselves to work at understanding his music in a way that audiences had perhaps never worked at understanding music before."[24] Those efforts were reflected in numerous reviews of unprecedented length published in leading musical journals, which at the time were broadly read by the literate musical public.[25]

This same argument, though, could just as well be made about Beethoven's music from twenty years before. A few of his works from just after 1800, including the *Eroica* Symphony but also the piano variations that gave rise to its last movement and the Third Piano Concerto, received unusually lengthy reviews, and so did many of the works that followed. Of the *Eroica*, an anonymous writer in the *Allgemeine musikalische Zeitung* said that "the uniqueness and the rich content of the work seem to demand that above all we seriously examine its technical aspects and in this regard, as well as in regard to its related mechanical aspects, follow the composer step by step."[26] By contrast, a writer in *Der Freymüthige* two years earlier had said that one group of listeners "denies this work any artistic value and feels that it manifests a completely unbounded striving for distinction and oddity, which, however, has produced neither beauty nor true sublimity and power."[27] The style of Beethoven's middle period clearly inspired the same kind of bafflement—and the same kind of determined effort to understand it—as did his late style.

Furthermore, those who rose to the defense of the middle-period works were responding to almost exactly the same concerns that would later be raised about the late ones. Less sympathetic critics had found this music "bizarre" (a favorite barb from nearly the beginning of Beethoven's career), excessively long, and disorganized, making unreasonable demands of performers and listeners alike.[28] The only significant difference from the late period is that these perceived faults were not yet blamed on deafness.

What sets the late works off, then, is that they have always been understood through the prism of deafness, their faults and virtues alike attributed to the fact that the man who wrote them could not hear. This view of the late music would come to have dramatic repercussions for our understanding of Beethoven's entire oeuvre. Joseph Fröhlich, reviewing the Ninth Symphony for the journal *Caecilia* the year after Beethoven's death, made a suggestion that was unprecedented at the time but was later applied retroactively to a wide swath of Beethoven's earlier music: this symphony was Beethoven's musical autobiography, in which he expressed his resistance to the dramatic events that had overwhelmed his life and gave voice to his determination to find joy in the face of tragedy.[29] *Per aspera ad astra*—through bitterness to the stars—is an expressive arc that could just as easily be ascribed to Beethoven's Fifth Symphony, and frequently was by later writers. It may seem obvious that the last movement of that symphony answers the turmoil of the work's earlier movements with a powerful affirmative response. Interestingly, though, this was not noted when the symphony first appeared. E. T. A. Hoffmann, author of perhaps the most celebrated Beethoven review in history, described the finale as a return to the dark, foreboding mood of the symphony's opening. It was only when Beethoven was known to be deaf that his music—that of the middle period as well as that of the late period—could come to be seen as an affirmation in the face of adversity. Historians then squared the circle by appealing to the Heiligenstadt Testament of 1802, in which Beethoven conveyed his determination to keep writing music despite his growing depression and isolation. Deafness could now be seen as the primary creative force behind the entire last twenty-five years of Beethoven's life.

It is thus very hard to approach Beethoven's late works—or even many of his earlier ones—without preconceptions about the deaf composer and the nature of what he did. The assumption is often made that in this music Beethoven either overcame his handicap or tried to do so and failed. Beethoven himself did not claim to be engaging his deafness in his music, either in the Heiligenstadt Testament or in any other surviving writings. For those broadly familiar with Beethoven's music, though, there is probably no point in trying to walk back two hundred years of reception history and hear the late works simply "as music." Deafness will always be a salient part of Beethoven's biography.

For Beethoven, however, the story was a very different one from that told by later writers. Hearing loss had haunted him since his twenties, and there could scarcely have been a moment when he was unaware of it. There was no smooth arc to Beethoven's life, no upward trajectory like that outlined by Fröhlich. There was only steady, determined adaptation, as Beethoven sought not to redeem his life but to salvage his vocation. In this regard his story and Barbara's converge once again.

* 4 *
Deafness, Vocation, Vision

Vocation, it is said, is more than a career. A person's vocation may grow and develop, but it remains incontestable, compelling—internal rather than imposed. Beethoven's vocation was composing music; composing was the thread that bound his life together and made it a whole. In writing music after common sense decreed that he should stop, he was responding to that vocation. He didn't stop because he couldn't stop, and he couldn't stop because he was impelled by an unstoppable force to make music, even in the most dire circumstances imaginable. Continuing to compose did not make him a hero; some would even say it made him a fool. Certainly it shows in the starkest of terms who Ludwig van Beethoven understood himself to be.

Nursing was Barbara's job, but she defined her vocation not by her work but by her relationships with others. She had longed to be a wife and a mother, and when she lost her first husband and her baby within weeks of each other, her work as a nurse was no consolation. After she and I learned she had a uterine septum that made it impossible for her to carry a baby past nine weeks, we unhesitatingly spent thousands of dollars on treatment that was not covered by insurance. Jennifer's birth in December 1991 and Jeremy's a little over two years later were no less miraculous than Beethoven writing the Ninth Symphony while unable to hear. Both outcomes show that vocation does not acknowledge limits; wherever possible, it finds a way beyond them.

When she went deaf in the right ear in 2000, Barbara stopped working as a nurse; one good ear was not enough to take blood pressures and perform other critical tasks, and her problems with balance and the visual aphasia would have ruled it out in any case. Her challenge now was not to lose her vocation; everything possible had to be done to maintain the social connections that gave meaning and structure to her life. The effort to do so flew in the face of the devastating social isolation that deafness can produce.

Both Barbara and Beethoven felt the full force of that isolation, but it is important to note that it is not a universal experience for those unable to hear. In fact, many Deaf people today find that their shared experience of deafness creates a rich sense of community. The importance of that community does much to explain the deep resistance to cochlear implants among the Deaf. Like oralism—the movement that historically aimed to teach deaf people to speak and to integrate them into the hearing community—cochlear implants pose a threat to those whose main way of connecting with others is sign language. If enough people get implants, especially as children, and are encouraged to use them instead of learning to sign, the signing Deaf community could face a very real existential threat.

But Barbara also felt threatened: her link with the hearing world disappeared overnight, and her vocation—which she had always defined by her relationships with others: mother, wife, daughter, nurse—threatened to disappear with it. It could be argued that both she and Beethoven would have been better off joining a close-knit and supportive community rather than trying to "go it alone." But by making the decisions they did, they were not turning their backs on community and vocation; they were reaching for both in what they believed to be the best way possible. Barbara chose not to learn sign language but to rely on technology, lipreading, and writing to understand others. She made that choice because it seemed to offer the shortest and most promising route back into the kind of community she knew. Our family stretched in new directions to try to help her, and she also sought out new paths on her own. In the twelve years that remained to her, about as many years as Beethoven's late period, she experienced a sudden, devastating blow that Beethoven did not: whereas his hearing declined gradually and inexorably, the onset of total deafness for her was shockingly abrupt.

⁂

The events of that week in June 2003 are still vivid in my mind. They jolted my life and Barbara's like a shifting fault line, leaving scars in the earth, roads buckled and deformed, familiar landmarks crumbling or dislocated. Sitting at lunch at a restaurant while we waited for the results of tests done in the emergency room that first morning, the children and I absorbed, without quite believing, that anything we wanted to say to Barbara had to be written down—and that this might be the new permanent shape of reality. We watched others ordering, eating, and conversing and understood with brutal clarity that they were living in safe space on ground that had not shifted beneath them, while we were teetering over an abyss they could not see. They might notice us writing to Barbara, but they had no idea we were still growing accustomed to the aftershocks of her sudden deafness.

Driving to Asheville, we met my mother and her husband for dinner and extended our hands to them across this ruined landscape. Then they took Jennifer and Jeremy to Knoxville with them while Barbara and I returned to Spartanburg on our own. We traveled a mangled highway, exploring without directions while other drivers calmly passed, indifferent to our plight.

As the next week went by and the children stayed with my mother, we developed a working routine. The legal pads began to fill up with my side of every conversation, from the most routine ("Are you ready for lunch?") to the most challenging ("What do we do next if the treatment doesn't work?"). It was hard work to communicate this way. Barbara could say whatever she wanted to, but she had no sense of the volume of her voice and frequently shouted in public, to the discomfiture of those around her. I had to take the time to write everything down, then hand her the pad so she could read it and respond. Conversation at meals was doubly awkward because I had to stop eating for extended intervals in order to carry on my half of the exchange. If we were walking somewhere together, we would both have to stop in order for me to say anything. This wasn't just a change in the way we talked to each other; it required a reorientation of our sense of time and space and how we communicated within them.

When this all got to be too difficult—which it frequently did—we would go to the computer. With my pianist's fingers I could type my thoughts at a much faster rate than I could write them longhand, and Barbara could read them as they scrolled across the screen and respond immediately. This way we could have something resembling a normal conversation, and the relief I felt at being able to do so looms large in my memories of those first few weeks. So does my anguish at doing something as simple as turning on the television and realizing that mere days ago my wife could have heard the speech, the music, and the sound effects, but that she might never do so again.

Speaking with longtime friends in Spartanburg before moving to Texas was unimaginably awkward. People didn't know what to say to Barbara, or if they did they had trouble putting it into words. So we focused on getting ready to leave. Much of the next month was consumed with doing expensive deferred maintenance on our house. We were ceaselessly overrun by contractors installing new carpet and wallpaper. While they worked, we packed, and finally we supervised the loading of nine years' worth of our lives into a moving truck, then painted the walls in several rooms a neutral white, effectively erasing our personalities from our home.

In the middle of this ordeal, the fateful road trip. In Waco a realtor spent a day driving us to houses that matched our needs and price range. We toured each of them in turn, Barbara often leaning on me for support due to her compromised balance. Every time something important was said that was not visually obvious, I had to write it down, while also videotaping the interiors for future reference. One of the strengths of our marriage was that we usually agreed on important things without much discussion; we both knew which house we wanted right away and made an offer on it that evening. I had to handle the details from the phone in our hotel room while Barbara watched my lips move. We firmed up the details and revisited the house the next day, then flew to Atlanta, where the children were waiting with Barbara's parents this time, and drove them back to Spartanburg to resume the move.

⁛

Sometime in July we got our first break. We received a call from an audiologist at Baylor who wanted to work with Barbara. She told us about the pocket talker, a device that she thought might help us, so only days after arriving in Waco we were in her office

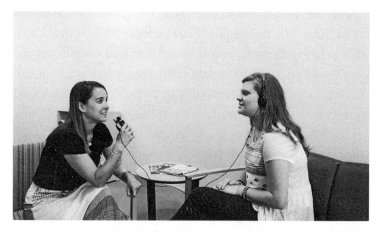

FIGURE 1. Carrie Drew (left) of the Baylor Speech-Language and Hearing Clinic demonstrates the use of the pocket talker in conversation.

learning how to use one. The pocket talker is a low-tech hearing aid (fig. 1). The sound it provides is not very refined but can be turned up to extremely high volumes. It consists of a box about the size of a pack of cigarettes with a small microphone protruding from the top. Instead of being worn on the body, it is handed directly to the speaker, while a cord connects it to a set of headphones. Thus the speaker and listener are physically joined. The microphone cannot simply be placed between them; the speaker has to hold it a few inches from his or her mouth. If it is held too far away, the sounds do not register. If it is held too close, they are distorted beyond recognition. If it is placed directly in front of the speaker's mouth, the sounds also don't register properly; it needs to be held down at about a 30-degree angle. At least this was our experience. Your mileage, we came to understand, may vary.

We had already ascertained that Barbara had a tiny amount of residual hearing in her right ear: 3 percent according to one test. In normal circumstances that ear was still practically useless. Only sounds of smoke-alarm volume would register at all, and even those sounded faint. In a soundproof booth she could occasionally identify a consonant. Outside the booth she could barely do that, even with the pocket talker blasting the sounds into her headphones. So she worked on speech recognition in her sessions with the audiologist, carefully listening to simple words and trying to learn to distinguish them.

Outside the sessions we quickly realized that she understood my voice better than most others and had particular difficulty hearing people whose voices were unfamiliar to her. Somewhat to our surprise, it did not help for me to speak loudly. Even though the pocket talker was conveying my voice to her at very high volume, she could understand me best when I spoke into it at a quiet, conversational level. This resonates with the experience of Beethoven, who reportedly could understand his friend and student Archduke Rudolph through his ear trumpets better than anybody else because of his "gentle voice."[1] Barbara could also understand me better when she looked directly at me as we spoke, although at first neither of us realized that this was because she was reading my lips.

Unfortunately, the pocket talker was practically useless when it came to music perception. Its inability to pick up sound coming from any distance away placed Barbara in a very small shell. She could not hear a public speaker or a live performance of anything. At home she heard nothing when I played the piano or the stereo. Even if I sang directly into the microphone, she heard no pitch variation. "It all sounds like a monotone," she said. Apparently the pocket talker was designed to convey and amplify the phonemes that are the basic components of speech, not the minute pitch variations that convey nuance and meaning and that are also the foundation of music. Using it, Barbara heard speech at a very rudimentary level, and she heard music not at all.

The most productive experiences occurred at church, where

there was a sound system that allowed hearing aids to connect to a portable receiving device. We found that hitching this device to the pocket talker allowed Barbara to follow parts of the service that were printed in the bulletin, and sometimes to hear enough of the sermon to get an idea of what it was about. These were incredible gifts, but music still eluded us. When we sang a hymn I would disconnect the pocket talker from the sound system, which conveyed only muddy noise, and sing directly into the microphone. If it was a hymn with which Barbara was familiar, she would try to keep up with me and would often come close. She watched me for cues, and the tactile memory in her vocal cords came to her aid and allowed her to sing the tune quite recognizably. Unfortunately she was often about a semitone off pitch, producing a discordant clash of which she was completely unaware. I would sometimes point out to Barbara afterward that she had been painfully out of tune, and after some initial trepidation she learned to say: "I don't care. I'm proud I can sing and I'm going to do it as loud and as off-key as ever you like. I refuse to be ashamed." I learned to agree with her, and to take pride in her singing as well.

It turned out, furthermore, that not only could she sing; almost unbelievably, she was also capable of learning new music. Barbara had always insisted that she couldn't read music. I was never sure what she meant by this. She knew what quarter notes and half notes were. She understood sharps and flats, time signatures, bar lines, and score notation. She could pick up at least a simple new piece in choir on Wednesday night and learn the alto part well enough to sing it on Sunday morning. Still, she insisted she couldn't read music. What she meant, I always suspected, was that she couldn't sight sing. Like a lot of people—probably the majority of people—she couldn't pick up a piece she hadn't heard before and sing it from the written notes without somebody else first singing or playing it for her.

Nevertheless, she managed to begin learning a new liturgy during the time she was using the pocket talker. Marty Haugen's *Now the Feast and Celebration* is an upbeat, folksy composition that makes no great demands on a congregation, but we had never heard it before moving to Texas. Our new church used it every other week, and the unison melodic line was always printed in the bulletin. Thus Barbara was able not just to hear me singing it through the pocket talker but to see the shape of the music as well. By the end of that first fall in Waco she was singing along and was getting many of the intervals right, even if she still didn't necessarily sing on pitch. Through some combination of tactile memory, eyesight, and extremely limited hearing, she was able to import new musical information and learn from it. This was the first of many experiences we had suggesting that music perception can work in ways we don't understand and transcend the arbitrary limits we tend to place on it.

In many ways the pocket talker was analogous to Beethoven's ear trumpets. Like them, it required a physical link between speaker and listener. As primitive as it seemed, it also avoided one of the most common problems reported by people using modern hearing aids: excessive amplification of background noise. Such amplification would later become a problem with the cochlear implants as well, but for the time being we could converse just as easily in public as we could in private—which is to say, not easily at all, but we were grateful for even this crumb of normalcy. After I started teaching we met regularly for lunch at restaurants near Baylor, where we would sit directly across from each other and use our mouths, eyes, and ears to communicate. Much of my side of the conversation was probably audible to others due to the volume coming from Barbara's headphones. Still, this was a vast improvement over half-written exchanges. I was relieved of the burden of having to write everything down, and Barbara had the satisfaction of being able to hear, even if in a very limited way.

Group conversation was a much bigger challenge; here we continually ran up against an obstacle in human nature that appeared to be bigger than the technology we were using. In theory it should be easy for a small group of people to sit at a table or in a circle and pass a microphone around. All that was necessary was for each person to pick up the pocket talker before beginning to speak. In practice, though, people would start neglecting to do this less than five minutes into the conversation. The more spontaneous a conversation became, the more likely they were to forget. As they began to focus on what they wanted to say next or on responding to what others had said, their attention shifted from the how of the conversation—picking up the microphone before speaking—to the what: jumping in and making their points before somebody else had a chance to speak. Furthermore, while people understood that it was necessary to speak slowly and clearly for Barbara to have a fighting chance of understanding, they would forget to do so almost immediately. We never once succeeded in having an extended group talk with the pocket talker.

These problems occurred even in groups sponsored by Marriage Encounter, an organization dedicated to promoting communication within marriage and community among married couples. We had been involved with Marriage Encounter for years, and after Barbara lost the hearing in her right ear and stopped working as a nurse we had begun to serve as presenters at their weekend retreats. This was one of the ways Barbara still sought to fulfill her vocation, and I was glad to be able to help her. As presenters we had to mingle with the other couples on the retreat and answer questions. This was a challenge for Barbara but not an insuperable one, especially with me there to facilitate.

When we tried to break into the Marriage Encounter network in Texas, though, we were stymied by the awkwardness of the pocket talker and others' inability to work around it. That awkwardness continued after Barbara later received her cochlear implant. Two months after hookup—the universal term of CI users for the activation of their implant—this is how she described the experience on Clarion, a Yahoo users' group for implant recipients in which she was a regular participant:

> Is it ever realistic to hope to obtain the ability to hear in groups? I know it has only been 2 months since I was hooked up and I am getting impatient. But my husband and I have been involved in Marriage Encounter as a presenting couple for nearly 3 years now. We, of course, have not presented since I went deaf. When we moved to Texas in August, I was so happy to be hooked up with another ME group. I really thought once I had my implant, I would again be able to participate. Last night, after attending the second presenters' meeting since hook up, I realized I could not hear them well enough even to follow the subject line. It quite depressed me. When, if ever, will I be able to hear in a group setting? I know everyone is different. I just need some idea to help me to cope better.[2]

Barbara left one meeting after another frustrated and in tears, and we finally decided the effort was counterproductive and gave up. The social isolation of deafness was too strong to be overcome by the best human intentions. I recount this not to impugn Marriage Encounter, an organization I respect, but to show the implacable nature of what both Barbara and Beethoven were up against.

Our family life, too, presented incalculable challenges. Our children were eleven and nine, and the dynamics of communicating with their mother in writing never quite sank in with them. Usually they would tell me what they wanted to say, and I would write it down for her. When we got the pocket talker they would mumble into it instead of speaking clearly. After I began teaching at Baylor they largely ignored Barbara when they were alone with her. I would come home at dinnertime, and they would immediately bombard me with stories about their day and questions about their homework. I hurt for Barbara, whom they had chosen to leave out of all this. Just as Beethoven feared the loss of his vocation for music, so she feared—and in part experienced—the loss of her vocation as a mother. Addressing this loss and ameliorating it was something all four of us would continue to struggle with in the years to come.

The same problems with group communication occurred when we tried using conversation books, only here the natural resistance level was even greater. A pad, not simply a microphone, had to be passed to each person who had something to say, then passed back to Barbara to read. Of course, in order to keep the conversation going it would also have to be read by everybody else present or spoken out loud. In the latter case, it was natural for the speaker to take advantage of the faster pace of speech and elaborate. Instead of saying "Do you need something from the store?" he or she would say, "I need to go to the store to get some groceries, so I asked if I could pick up anything for her." In this way Barbara was doubly excluded from the flow of the conversation: first, because people neglected to write things down, and second, because even what was written down was often rudimentary.[3]

The relevance of this to Beethoven is clear. Those who write about the conversation books often casually present them as "one half of the conversation" or as "a one-sided record of the way Beethoven interacted with others after he became deaf, from which everything he said is missing." This they clearly were not. Rather, they were a desperate compromise that might at times have paradoxically left him feeling more isolated than ever. We should not expect the surviving entries to read like half of a spoken conversation, and when multiple people were involved, the resemblance to a normal conversation in all likelihood decreased sharply.

For Beethoven this was the end of the road. Conversation books and ear trumpets were as close as he could come to normal conversation. Obviously they were lifesavers; without them, he would have been even more drastically alone. If a cochlear implant had been available to him, though, it seems reasonable to imagine that he would have tried it.

⁂

The possibility of an implant was first raised to Barbara and me at Duke in 2000. Until then we knew little about them. I remembered reading an article in a magazine written by a woman whose deaf husband had received an implant; his ability to hear with it was presented as a miracle of modern medicine. The idea, I understood, was simple in concept but difficult to pull off. A microphone picked up sounds and relayed them to an array of electrodes situated inside the cochlea, the innermost part of the ear, so that they could be received by the auditory nerve and register in the brain as sound. The result might not be quite the same as the way things "actually" sounded, but it was close enough to transform the lives of the relatively small number of profoundly deaf patients who had received implants. Now they could hear well enough to converse with their families, hold jobs, and perhaps even enjoy music.[4]

Every one of these assumptions would turn out to be problematic, but we didn't have a chance to find that out in 2000 because of an even more immediate problem: money. Furthermore, we were led to believe that research on the regeneration of the hair cells in the cochlea was sufficiently advanced that we might expect to see it happen during our lifetimes. The hair cells are the ear's own mechanism for receiving sound. Despite their name they are actually nerve cells, and like other nerve cells, when they are damaged they don't regenerate. This is why nearly everybody sustains hearing loss as part of the aging process. The hair cells die and they are not replaced. As I write this I am aware that at fifty-nine I don't hear as well as I used to, though this is more of an annoyance than a real problem. By the time I'm seventy I expect to be missing a lot more, as do most people of that age. Solving this problem would benefit not only those with sensorineural deafness but virtually all older adults as well.

So in 2000 we were encouraged to sit tight and not put our hopes in a cochlear implant. But this changed almost immediately after Barbara lost the hearing in her left ear. The focus now shifted to figuring out if she was a good candidate for an implant. The first step was a CT scan of her auditory nerve to make sure it was still capable of transmitting the signals past the cochlea. The results were encouraging. Before we moved to Texas we found that implant surgeries were being done in Dallas and San Antonio, and since Dallas was closer to Waco we decided to go through the office of Dr. Robert Owens, who worked, appropriately, at the Baylor Medical Center. (At that time the Baylor Hospital in Dallas was still affiliated with Baylor University.) Once medical necessity and feasibility were established, our new insurance approved the procedure, and implantation was scheduled for the week before Thanksgiving 2003.[5]

Cochlear implantation is normally an outpatient surgery. Because we had a hundred-mile drive back to Waco, Barbara was kept in the hospital overnight. The next day she was released wearing something like a turban around her head and sent home to heal. She still heard nothing, and her tinnitus grew worse.

Over the next week my mother came to visit and helped me cook Thanksgiving dinner. Jennifer turned twelve. The semester at Baylor ended the week after that, and I gave my first final exams in my new job, then launched into the usual end-of-semester grading marathon. Still, with Christmas fast approaching, Barbara and I were focused on only one thing: activation, which would take place on December 19, my forty-eighth birthday. It is hard to convey how much was riding on that event. Until it happened, there was no guarantee the implant would work at all. Failures were not unheard of. On the other hand, we had heard stories of people whose implants were turned on and who were immediately able to talk on the phone and hear music. Anything seemed possible, but at least we thought we would have an answer.

The two hours we spent at the audiologist's office in Dallas were an extraordinary and haunting experience. It began when the "audie" (as we learned to call her) placed the external audio processor behind Barbara's ear and hooked it up to her computer. It was now connected to Barbara's head through a magnet, which bonded to the metal plate on the implant beneath her skull, but there was as yet no external microphone. Any sound Barbara was going to hear at this point would emerge from the computer and would not in any way be heard by anyone else in the room.

Watching the computer screen, I could see the sixteen audio channels, each of which fed one of the electrodes in Barbara's cochlea. I could see the sound she was receiving even though I could not hear it. The audie proceeded to "map" each of the channels in turn, raising the sound gradually until it reached a point where Barbara found it comfortable: neither too loud nor too soft. This was the first time she had heard anything in her left ear since June, and I expected to see her face light up with pleasure as soon as she had conclusive proof that the implant was working.

It didn't go that way. She simply methodically responded, indicating with hand motions when the sounds—she said they sounded like organ notes—were loud enough. Once all of the channels had been mapped, the audie turned on the processor's internal microphone. For the first time in months, Barbara had the opportunity to understand speech. Once again, I expected surprise and delight but was met with something more like confusion. My voice, which was the first thing she tried to hear, baffled her. After being used to the pocket talker, she could barely understand what I was saying. Even though it was clear the implant was working, she was disappointed. She had expected something better than this confusing jumble of sounds.

Things improved only slightly when the audie connected the "T-Mic," a new invention from Advanced Bionics, the company that manufactured her implant, consisting of an external microphone that can actually be placed inside the ear. Some more mapping followed as the audie tried to maximize the quality of the sound Barbara was able to hear. She then encouraged us to wander around the hospital and experiment with talking to each other. So we went to the cafeteria and got a snack and talked. Or, rather, we tried to talk, because it turned out to be much more of a struggle than it had been with the pocket talker. But we had strict instructions to put the pocket talker away and never use it again. The goal now was to get used to communicating with the implant, and it was clear that it was going to be a slow and difficult learning process.

The outermost portion of the cochlea, where the electrodes

had been attached, contains the hair cells that register the highest pitches, so the impulses from the electrodes naturally registered as high pitches as well. Immediately after activation, most voices, including mine, sounded to Barbara like squawky cartoon characters. Far from being pleased with what she was hearing, she was clearly disillusioned and discouraged.

Within days, though, voices started to come down in pitch; soon I was sounding like Michael Jackson rather than Daffy Duck. Eventually my voice came to sound something like she remembered.

All of these "sounds," meanwhile, were being conveyed to the implant by means of an external processor that fit behind Barbara's ear and connected to her head magnetically (fig. 2). At the time she received her implant, this behind-the-ear (BTE) processor was a new development. Previous cochlear implant recipients had received a body-worn processor that was

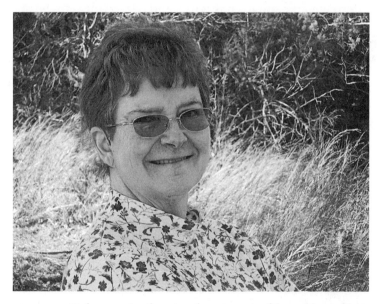

FIGURE 2. Barbara wearing the external components of the cochlear implant.

considerably larger. The "T-mic" that Barbara received was also brand new, and it was designed to take advantage of the sound-catching structure of her outer ear. The signals it picked up, after being "processed," were relayed through the magnets inside and outside her head to the implant, where the signals were modified even further before being conveyed to the electrodes. What happened to the signals in between was, to say the least, complex. The sounds picked up by the microphone had to be translated into digital code that would tell the electrodes when to fire and compressed into the sixteen channels along which that firing could take place. The volume had to be adjusted constantly so that quiet sounds were audible but loud sounds weren't overwhelming. Digital information had to be relayed at a mind-boggling pace. The process operated by a program called Hi-Res, which, like the T-mic, was new enough to be in the experimental phase.

Also experimental was the strategy by which the processor interpreted the sounds it received and relayed them to the implant. Two different processing strategies were available, and both of them were programmed into Barbara's processor. The paired strategy stimulated two electrodes at a time and thus operated at a faster pace. The sequential strategy stimulated one electrode at a time, so each one had to fire before any of them got a chance to fire again. This seemed to work better for Barbara, so we stuck with it.

The processor also came with four rechargeable batteries, each of which would last for about four hours before suddenly expiring. The time varied, because the more sound Barbara heard, the more quickly the battery would wear out. It took all four to get through a typical day, and then they needed to be recharged while Barbara was sleeping. This meant that at most she could hear for about sixteen hours. If she stayed up late, she became deaf again, and of course at night she still heard nothing.

The implant had worked; we no longer needed to be dogged by the fear of permanent deafness. Nevertheless, when we left the office for the drive back to Waco, we were both disappointed. If we hadn't had the pocket talker to communicate with for the previous four months, this would have seemed like the miracle it indeed was. Barbara, we were assured, was doing quite well to be able to understand any words at all; many implant recipients hear only undifferentiated sounds for the first several weeks after hookup. But we had to struggle to communicate on the way home. She could hear me only if I looked directly at her so she could read my lips, and of course I couldn't do that while I was driving. We stopped at a restaurant for dinner (since it was my birthday), and the more crowded it got, the less she understood. By the end of dinner I was back to writing everything down for her. On the other hand, she was able to hear background noise, like the waitress walking by our table, and was even aware that there was music playing, although she couldn't tell what it was. Most remarkable of all, I no longer had to talk directly into a microphone for her to understand.

Still, we went to bed that night tired and a little depressed. We had had visions of Barbara being able to talk on the phone the first day (as one new friend of hers could) and perhaps being able to listen to Christmas songs on the radio. None of that was even close. This was not the dramatic step forward we had been hoping for.

But things improved rapidly. A few days later we flew to California to spend Christmas with Barbara's family. While we were there, about ten days after activation, we finally had the experience we had wanted on the drive home from Dallas.

⁙

We had gone out to dinner with a large group of Barbara's family members. This was a frustrating experience because the loud restaurant and the rapid conversation had left Barbara feeling isolated. After dinner we drove home by ourselves in one of her parents' cars. We talked about the implant and the fact that sounds were still arriving in selective, limited ways. We talked about the changes that had occurred in the area since we had lived there: the endless growth gobbling up what had been empty space when we first met. We talked about the days before the children were born, when we were free to go to movies or out to dinner on the spur of the moment.

Suddenly it dawned on us that this was the first real conversation we had had since before we moved to Texas. I was driving, and Barbara sat to my right with her implanted ear pointing toward me. She was hearing nearly every word I said.

That didn't mean we could now talk normally, of course. It meant that in a closed environment with limited background noise she could understand my voice, with which she was intimately familiar, most of the time. Participating in groups, talking with strangers, conversing in public, listening to music, and interacting with our children would continue to pose huge challenges. The following June, Barbara would share this advice with new implant recipients:

> The voice you're used to the most will be the voice you can understand the best. In my case it is my husband's voice. I can even talk to him fairly well on the phone, occasionally not even asking him to repeat something! But it's different with every single person I talk to. My brain has to get used to their voice so I can understand it. My doctor tells me it will take 1 year and possibly much more to get to a point where I can hear things quite well.[6]

In fact, it would take much longer than that; hearing "quite well" was an elusive goal that she never actually attained, even after receiving an implant in her other ear and upgrading her external processors. But our progress was still deeply satisfying, both emotionally and intellectually.

Years later I had an experience that, in retrospect, helped me understand what this time was like for Barbara. It was a quiet afternoon, and I was sitting in a reclining chair in my office trying to catch a nap when a strange sound I couldn't place began to intrude. I thought I heard two quick, buzzerlike noises in quick succession, over and over again; they were mildly alarming because I couldn't connect them to any idea of a source. Then suddenly it dawned on me: I was listening to a car alarm, its sound distorted by distance and by traveling through the ground in order to register in my basement office. With this realization came an abrupt transformation of the sound itself. It no longer sounded like a buzzer. Now that I had identified it as a car alarm, it sounded completely different: it was clearly a horn, and I was no longer capable of hearing it as a buzz.

Barbara apparently went through this process over and over again during the first months she had the implant. As I observed it I began to change the way I think about sensory perception. It is natural to assume that sounds and sights are external to us and that our senses enable us to hear and see them. The idea that the mind has to format reality before it can perceive anything at all might make sense to an epistemologist schooled on Immanuel Kant, but to the rest of us the distinction can easily sound like abstruse nitpicking. At least it can until your experience confirms it. As the year 2004 unfolded and Barbara's implant was repeatedly remapped, it became clear that the really significant changes were taking place not in the software but in her brain. The squawky, high-pitched sounds that she heard when I spoke to her after activation made physiological sense; only the outer part of her cochlea, which registers high pitches, was being stimulated by the implant, since this was as far as the electrodes could safely be inserted. Only a limited range of pitch information was being conveyed by the processor: sixteen channels in all. No wonder I sounded like a cartoon character.

Barbara wanted to hear me sound like myself, though, so her brain began working on making me sound that way. This was not a conscious process. She didn't tell her brainstem and auditory cortex to shift from Daffy to Robin. The shift happened passively—not all at once but in gradual stages: first Daffy Duck, then Michael Jackson, then a deeper, generic male voice, and finally something that she could identify as being me. Whether my voice sounded exactly the same to her as it had before she lost her hearing is not clear; there is no objective metric for determining such things. What mattered was that there was now a voice she heard as Robin that fit into the Robin-shaped framework in her head.

Gradually other voices began to fit into similar frameworks, and she could hear the speakers as individuals too. Barking dogs and airplane noises got sorted into their own defined categories. The piano began to sound like a piano to her long before she could hear the notes as discrete pitches. In fact, when I first played her a single note she said it sounded like an entire chord; her brain was apparently registering each of the first few overtones as separate pitches. This gradually subsided, but a few months after activation we attended a piano recital of music by Beethoven and Brahms. We sat close to the stage, and Barbara reported that she heard the music clearly, but it all sounded modern. In other words, the timbres and rhythms were coming through, but the pitches hadn't yet sorted themselves out.

Throughout that first year we drove back to Dallas at least once a month for new mappings. We began to experiment with new programming strategies. The processor allowed for three different settings, and both could be adjusted for loudness and input dynamic range (IDR), or the amount of sound that was delivered at once. Increasing IDR meant that Barbara could hear more background noise; decreasing it allowed her to focus on a single voice. As with most things involving the cochlear implant, though, it wasn't really that simple. As Barbara grew used to hearing with the implant, she was able to tolerate more volume and a wider IDR, and it became clear that she needed them. What had sounded adequate after the previous mapping would quickly come to sound too soft and indistinct. Thus these settings had to be constantly readjusted as the auditory circuits in her brain rapidly redrew themselves. At one point we found that despite the increasing amount of sound Barbara was able to tolerate—or perhaps because of it—she heard better when only eight of the sixteen channels were being activated, so for a while this became our default programming strategy.

We eventually settled on three different settings: one for everyday use, one for loud public places in which IDR was turned down to control background noise, and one for public events like concerts and lectures in which it was turned up in order to bring in as much sound as possible. We referred to the last of these as the "music" setting, since it was supposed to allow Barbara to hear more at live concerts. Oddly, though, her most successful experiences listening to music were usually with the everyday setting. This was a reflection of a reality that we often tried to ignore: the programming strategies on which the cochlear implant operated were designed to facilitate the understanding of speech, not music. Whatever musical benefits we got were not part of the package. There was no way to intentionally make music sound better, and every situation was different. In 1815 Beethoven, reflecting on the technology available to him at the time, noted in his diary that "one should have different [ear trumpets] in the room for music, speech, and also for halls of various sizes."[7] Just like Beethoven, Barbara was learning that hearing functions differently in different situations, and like Beethoven's friend Mälzel, who designed a series of ear trumpets for him, her audiologists were experimenting with different solutions with mixed success.

Because my job gives me access to a lot of free classical concerts, we continued to attend regularly. A performance by a chamber group, including violin, cello, and horn, produced an intriguing realization. Once again we sat near the front, so Barbara could not only hear but also watch the instrumentalists and coordinate what she saw them doing with the sounds they produced. By focusing on the cellist, she was able to pick out the sounds of that instrument and distinguish them from those of the horn and the higher-pitched violin. As soon as she began to do that, the other instruments disappeared. They didn't just fade into the background—she could no longer hear them at all, even though the cello was registering clearly. Eventually— several months down the road—she would get to the point where she could focus this way on two instruments at the same time.

I still have very little idea of what Barbara was actually hearing during these concerts. The classical music repertory is vast, so most of the music being played was not familiar to her. Classical pieces can be lengthy—a single movement may run ten minutes or more—and they rarely present something as easy to follow as a simple melody and accompaniment. But melody is exactly what Barbara was hoping to hear, and occasionally there would be breakthroughs. A few months after activation she was working in the kitchen and figured out, on her own, that Jennifer was playing Offenbach's *Can-Can* on the violin in the next room. Barbara was moved to tears both because she was able to hear it at all and because she was able to identify the tune. At the same time, it was hardly surprising that this particular tune caused the breakthrough. The *Can-Can* is a catchy melody with a distinctive profile that is familiar to nearly everybody, even if they don't know that it is technically the "Infernal Galop" from the operetta *Orpheus in the Underworld*. Like the memorable motifs that appear in many of Beethoven's works, it is the kind of thing that could easily fit onto a card in the mental Rolodex, next to the sound of the neighbor's dog. The entire cello part of a Brahms piano trio simply could not be heard and categorized in the same way. But Barbara told me she was hearing enough to hold her interest, so we continued to attend.

A few things were clear from these experiences, as unpromising as they might seem. Rhythm was the easiest musical element for Barbara to recognize; percussive timbres[8]—including the piano—and wind timbres registered best. Short, highly recognizable melodic profiles seemed to play a crucial role in stimulating her auditory cortex. Visual cues were extremely important as well.

It is tempting to use these brief observations to make some preliminary guesses about Beethoven, hearing loss, and creativity. That Beethoven often wrote highly rhythmic music is obvious, as is the fact that he explored the timbral possibilities of the piano in novel ways. As his deafness grew, his use of motifs— short, highly recognizable melodic profiles—began to define his style to an unprecedented extent. There is no more familiar cultural icon in music than the first four notes of Beethoven's Fifth Symphony. The rhythm and melodic profile even look distinctive on paper. It is seemingly a perfect fit for the mental "Rolodex" in which musical memories are stored. Its powerful, distinctive rhythm means that its relentless reiterations can be felt throughout the body. When Barbara and I traveled to

Dallas in September 2007 for a preview of Advanced Bionic's new Harmony 120 processor, I brought a recording of the Fifth Symphony on my iPod so it could be fed directly into her CI through a patch cord. Those of us who were observing her heard nothing—there was no actual music to hear—but it was clear that she was having a powerful musical experience from the very first notes. The Harmony uses a technique called current steering to stimulate two electrodes simultaneously, theoretically allowing the user to hear a wider range of pitches than is possible when only one is stimulated at a time.[9] We would later be disappointed in the results, which turned out not to be as good at improving music perception as we had hoped. When she listened to the Fifth Symphony, though, Barbara was initially enchanted.[10]

The rhythmic drive of the Fifth Symphony is so effective because it is both powerful and erratic. As Toscanini conveyed with his body language, the pauses are present just as much as the notes are. It is clear from Beethoven's manuscript that he felt the music this way too, since the rests in measures 1 and 3 are set squarely in the middle, squeezing the three eighth notes into a portion of the remaining space on the right. The rest on the downbeat is the essential musical event of these measures. As the music continues, the rests regularly return, punctuated by dramatic crescendos and hammering repetitions of the central motive, which can be heard in the later movements as well.

Still, Beethoven's music is hardly easy for someone with hearing loss to absorb. As he grew deafer, his works became longer, his use of motifs more subtle and complex. His goal was clearly not to produce music that was easy for a deaf person to follow.

Or was it? The recent edition of Landsberg 6, the *Eroica* sketchbook, by Lewis Lockwood and Alan Gosman, makes a large portion of Beethoven's work on his pivotal Third Symphony visible both in facsimile and in transcription. These are sketches that Beethoven produced immediately after the Heiligenstadt crisis and in which he visibly struggled to put together his longest and most complex work to date. The symphony's first movement is dominated by a motif as easily recognizable as that of the Fifth, and like that later motif it is distinctive in appearance as well. It occupies two full measures in ¾ time. Each of those measures begins with a half note on the same pitch and continues with a quarter note. Beethoven, in his characteristic hand, wrote the quarter notes in a single gesture, as staffs with curves at the end instead of black note heads. To write the half notes, he picked up his pen and made a separate curl to the left of the main staff. Writing down each measure, in other words, required three separate strokes of Beethoven's pen, the first two dedicated to the half note on beats one and two and the third one to the quarter note on beat three. In the longer version of the motif, measure 3, containing three quarter notes, could also be written with three quick penstrokes, as could the dotted half note in measure 5, the dot occupying the notational equivalent of the third beat. For Beethoven, to set this music on paper was to feel its distinctive rhythm in his body (fig. 3).

As Lockwood and Gosman have observed, Beethoven then returned to this motif again and again in the long series of drafts he made for the first movement.[11] Sometimes it is only suggested by the appearance of its distinctive eighth-note accompaniment. Much more frequently, though, the motif appears in its own right, its unique profile highly visible amid the jumble of halfs, quarters, eighths, and sixteenth notes that fill up the remainder of the sketch pages. Beethoven often used it as a stand-in for other important thematic events. Its appearance, usually in the original key of E-flat, served "as a signal that he is not yet satisfied. The E♭ version ultimately serves

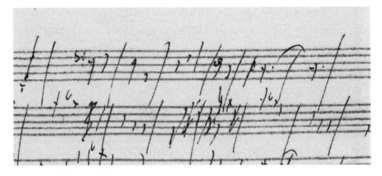

FIGURE 3. The top line of page 11 of Beethoven's sketchbook
Landsberg 6. Source: Lewis Lockwood and Alan Gosman,
eds., *Beethoven's "Eroica" Sketchbook: A Critical Edition*,
vol. 2 (Urbana: University of Illinois Press, 2013).

as a placeholder and reserves a musical space for a yet-to-be-
determined theme."[12] In the finished work something different usually occurs at these spots, but in the sketches it is near-
omnipresent.

Beethoven, in other words, was using a simple visual cue—
one that stood for a musically noteworthy event and was itself
grounded in his physical sense of time—to help consolidate
what would turn out to be one of the longest, most complex
musical structures yet written. Just like Barbara when she focused on watching the cellist and let the other instruments fade
out, he let his eyes take the lead. The movement's audible complexity was based on something he could see: something that
is still visible to anyone who cares to follow his path through
the pages of Landsberg 6.

* * *

Sight proved crucial to Barbara's enjoyment of music in other
ways as well. Although she frequently kept the radio on in the
car, she rarely heard anything as satisfying as the sudden rev-
elation of "Eight Days a Week." Even plugging a CD player

directly into her processor with a patch cord had indifferent results. When she attended a live performance, though, she could pick up on a wide variety of visual cues: the performers came on stage, took their positions, marked time, showed signs of emotion, and involved themselves physically in the act of making music. Others in the audience also paid attention and showed their appreciation. Jazz performances were among the best experiences we had together, not just because the music was rhythmic in a way Barbara could easily pick up on but because the performers were less inhibited, often standing when they had solos or otherwise calling attention to themselves, and because some in the audience sat less stiffly and occasionally got up and danced. Barbara described one such experience in one of her most ebullient Yahoo group posts.

> Tonight I went to a Jazz Ensemble concert with my husband. For the first time, even though my hearing music still has a long way to go to reach even near perfection level, I can honestly say I heard enough to thoroughly enjoy this concert!!!! Usually when I leave concerts, I tend to be a bit depressed because I haven't heard things to the "appreciation level," as I call it. Tonight, I left with a big grin on my face!!!! I didn't know if I'd ever be able to hear music this well again!!![13]

Although I am still not sure I understand how much or what she was hearing, I had no reason to doubt that for Barbara this performance was a major breakthrough. For both her and Beethoven, music was bigger than the sense of hearing alone.

Barbara's vocation, meanwhile, was something that continued to elude her even as she won a multitude of small victories. Talking with the children became easier as they grew older, though she rarely felt like she had the kind of natural back-and-forth with them that she had hoped for and expected. She could take them places in the car—an essential parenting task in today's world—but she missed one of the benefits of driving "Mom's taxi": the chance to converse with them while in transit. Hearing with a cochlear implant was hard mental work, and when she drove, her attention naturally had to be on the road. Dinner conversation, too, remained strained. Often she would start saying something on a new topic while somebody else was in the middle of a sentence, which reminded us that if she didn't know we were speaking she often didn't hear us at all. It seemed like she wasn't paying attention, but as with everything involving the implants, the truth was more complicated. The work involved in hearing us was apparently so great that she needed regular mental breaks. She compared the experience to having to spend all day conversing in a foreign language she didn't know very well. Anybody who has ever tried to do this will understand that there are times when the effort becomes too great and you have to allow the sounds to stop making sense in order to let your mind relax. Barbara had to work just as hard, if not harder, to understand people speaking her native language. Unlike a traveler in a foreign land, though, she had no way ever to return to her own country and listen fluently again. All she could do was temporarily turn her hearing "off."

One of her proudest accomplishments was completing the course of training for the Stephen Ministry at our church despite these challenges. Stephen Ministers are laypeople who visit with others in the congregation who are experiencing bereavement or loss. They go through a year of preparation to learn to become skilled and responsive listeners. Although Barbara still struggled to hear during these meetings, she stuck with it doggedly because she knew that listening was a special gift of hers, one that was not dependent on the functioning of her ears. Eventually she ministered to an elderly woman who was unable to attend church, and she became the eyes and ears of the congregation to her.

Jennifer played violin in the school orchestra all the way through middle school and high school and on into college, and played in a community youth orchestra as well. Jeremy sang in the Waco Boys' Choir and in a succession of school choirs, and also performed in regular piano and voice recitals as he came to an understanding of his own vocation for music. Barbara attended every single one of these performances, sitting close to the front where she could see and have at least a chance of hearing something as well. Afterward I would ask her how much she had been able to catch. The answer was almost always the same: "Hardly anything." Persistence and determination did not pay off, yet she continued to attend because she loved her children and knew her presence was important to them.

Looking back over those years, I understand that Barbara was a person of enormous courage who was sustained by hope and refused to surrender it. Life was often an unthinkable struggle for her as disappointments mounted and new challenges grew like weeds. Although she largely hid her frustration from others, there were many times when she told me she hated her life, hated being herself. Yet the story of calm, collected persistence that she presented to the world was not a lie. She did what she could and seemingly had no regrets about her efforts. Despite the often devastating setbacks, she learned to live within her limits, even when those limits were harsh and unfathomable. I and many others found this to be a gift, uniquely hers.

Two years before Barbara died, Jeremy's piano teacher—one of the pillars of Waco's music community—was diagnosed with a brain tumor. Characteristically, Barbara did not want to offer cheap encouragement by telling him her own story of survival. Instead she brought him a plate of Christmas cookies and visited with him for a while, inclining her stronger left ear toward him in the effort to hear him better. A few months later he was gone, having continued to teach almost to the end. Thus is the call of vocation heard through myriad human lives, often unremarkable but life-giving in ways small as well as large. To seek vocation requires patience. To answer it requires courage. Only by ignoring vocation can one be judged a failure.

* 5 *
The Artifacts of Deafness

Beethoven's response to his vocation can be seen not just in the music he produced after his hearing began to fail. It can also be understood through the abundance of physical objects that helped him remain musically active in the face of that enormous challenge. These include not just assistive devices, like his iconic ear trumpets, which he used only after his deafness became severe, but also the pianos and writing implements he had mastered years before. These he began to use in novel ways, and it is clear that they became more, not less, important to him as his perception of sound deteriorated.

Landsberg 6, the *Eroica* sketchbook, is not unique. Some of the most obvious adjustments Beethoven made after he began to lose his hearing can be seen throughout his sketches and manuscripts, which showed signs of ever more extensive planning and revision and became increasingly hard to read. He left behind an extraordinarily large number of sketches — more than exist for any previous composer or perhaps for any since. In them he made first drafts of his musical ideas, expanded on them, and experimented with ways of making them into finished works. He often compiled his sketches into collections, which have come to be known as sketchbooks, even though they consist of sheets of manuscript paper which Beethoven bound together himself. Some were desk sketchbooks, large enough that they did not leave his home except when he moved. Others were smaller "pocket" sketchbooks that Beethoven could carry around to jot down ideas whenever they occurred to him. Beethoven's sketches have fascinated admirers of his music since at least the late nineteenth century, when Gustav Nottebohm began publishing transcriptions and commentaries on them. However, those who wished to follow in Nottebohm's footsteps had a series of enormous hurdles to surmount. After Beethoven's death many of the sketches were separated from the collections into which the composer had bound them, and they scattered throughout the world. Those collections themselves passed through a variety of private hands, and many still bear the names of an international cast of previous owners: Kafka, de Roda, Wielhorsky, and Rolland, to name but a few. They are still dispersed so widely that it would be virtually impossible for one person to look at all of them directly.

Time has not stood still, however; the sketchbooks have been largely reconstructed and their chronological sequence established.[1] Systematic publications of facsimiles, commentaries, and transcriptions have helped to demystify some of the more important collections.[2] Many others can be viewed online, and good facsimiles of Beethoven manuscripts can also be found online or in print.[3] Thus anyone with the time and interest can look in great detail at the handwritten evidence of Beethoven's creative process.

And such a person is likely to find that evidence daunting. The appearance of many of the sketches and manuscripts is chaotic. Paper and ink seem to have collided in vast whorls of sprawling stems, bars, lines, clefs, slurs, and corrections. It's not easy to place yourself inside Beethoven's creative world.

At the same time, though, many of the sketches have a visual appeal that is hard to deny. Like abstract art, they invite

the eye to make connections that lie beneath the surface. Or
rather, like a medieval manuscript of music we can no longer
read, they present patterns that are visually intriguing in their
own right. Look, for example, at page 7 of Artaria 195, a late
sketchbook that is available in a sumptuous three-volume edition by William Kinderman. This page is the beginning of a
long section of the sketchbook devoted to the monumental "Et
vitam venturi saeculi" fugue that concludes the Credo of the
Missa Solemnis, Beethoven's great mass setting from his final
years (fig. 4).

The subject of the fugue looks distinctive; four stately half
notes in succession on the same pitch are followed by four
more that outline a descent by thirds. Thus if the initial pitch
falls on a line of the staff the others fall on lines as well, and likewise if the initial pitch falls on a space. Since the meter is 3/2
these four notes are split by a bar line, with the first pitch, the
upbeat, standing alone. As a result, the middle section of the
page, written in pen, is adorned by a very recognizable pattern.
Unlike some Beethoven sketches where writing is crammed
into every available space and the noteheads are tiny to non-
existent, these notes stand proudly on uncrowded space and
invite the eye to trace the shape they form. That shape is mir-
rored in the penciled lines at the bottom of the page, lighter in
color but spread out more widely and decorated by a counter-
subject in quarter notes.

As the sketches continue on the following pages, the distinctive subject can be seen again and again, floating serenely
through the surrounding chaos. Indeed, though many of the
passages Beethoven sketched do not appear in the finished
work, the sketches look much the way the music sounds. In a
fugue, a subject—usually short and highly recognizable—is repeated again and again while a complex musical tapestry flows
around it. Often it is combined with itself in ways that can be

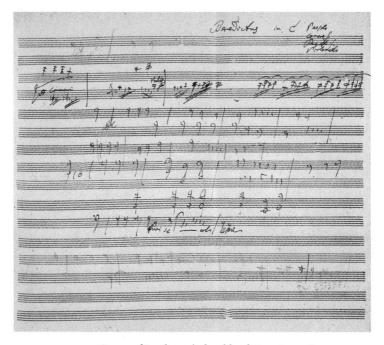

FIGURE 4. Page 7 of Beethoven's sketchbook Artaria 195. Source:
William Kinderman, ed., *Artaria 195: Beethoven's Sketchbook
for the "Missa Solemnis" and the Piano Sonata in E Major, Opus
109*, vol. 2 (Urbana: University of Illinois Press, 2003).

seen in the score as well as heard, particularly toward the end
as the composer "pulls out the stops." Beethoven's sketches cut
directly to the chase, allowing the subject to harmonize with itself visually before the musical elaboration even begins. This is
a fugue for the eyes, from which the one for the ears will eventually emerge. As this sketch demonstrates, the visual appeal of
fugal writing, in which short subjects can be repeatedly seen as
well as heard, helps to explain Beethoven's growing attraction
to this style in his late years.

Most Beethoven sketches do not show such a clear connection between the drafting on paper and the shape of music that
grew from it. Nevertheless, it has long been recognized that a
distinctive feature of Beethoven's sketching process is his use

of "continuity drafts," which show substantial portions of the finished work on a single staff, minus the details that will flesh them out but with the most essential musical content always visible. Beethoven probably learned this manner of working from Haydn, who referred to this stage of drafting as *Componieren*: the intermediate written stage between *Phantasieren*— improvising at the keyboard—and *Setzen*, writing down the finished work.[4] It was a way of laying out the work visually before it was completed, and Beethoven took it to unprecedented lengths. In their study of Landsberg 6, Lewis Lockwood and Alan Gosman found that while Beethoven was working on the *Eroica* he frequently folded pages of his sketchbook in a way that allowed him to view materials on distant pages simultaneously.[5] When he was working on the revisions of *Fidelio* in 1814, Beethoven complained to his librettist, "The way I am accustomed to writing, even in my instrumental music I always have the whole in view."[6] He apparently meant this literally. Having the whole in view was not just something he did in his head. It was something he did on paper.

The *Eroica*, begun immediately after the Heiligenstadt crisis in 1802, was a watershed. In this music the monumental scale that would characterize the works of Beethoven's middle, heroic period seems to have fully congealed, endowing instrumental music with new expressive power. The number of continuity drafts and the amount of page-folding Beethoven employed to arrive at that goal show that he was fully conscious of what he was doing and that he torqued his materials in ways that frequently allowed his eyes to take the lead.

Physical objects of all kinds were important to Beethoven's work as a composer, and a careful consideration of them yields many such intriguing clues about how he adjusted to his hearing loss. We must proceed with caution, though, because misconceptions also abound, particularly when it comes to Beethoven's use of the piano and his attitudes toward it.

The Ever-Changing Piano

There is a widely repeated story that after Beethoven began to lose his hearing, he removed the legs from his piano and placed it on the floor. A quick Google search will reveal many different versions of this legend, invariably presented as received knowledge and without documentation. The act of removing the legs is often described as violent: Beethoven is said to have hacked or sawed them off the instrument (what he did with the pedals is less clear). Afterward he could supposedly feel the piano's vibrations through the floor with his whole body, and this allegedly helped him hear and compose.

If Beethoven did these things, his experience would resonate with that of some other deaf musicians (Evelyn Glennie comes to mind) who have also felt music as vibration, affirming an essential continuity between the sense of hearing and that of touch. But where does the story come from? Its sole contemporary source is a letter from Bettina Brentano (later von Arnim). She visited Beethoven in Vienna and wrote of seeing "two or three pianos, all without legs and lying on the ground" in the front room of his apartment.[7] If she is to be believed—and her reminiscences have frequently been questioned because of their fanciful tone—Beethoven had multiple pianos in his possession in 1810. In any case Brentano's description is meant to point up his bad housekeeping: it also mentions unpacked trunks, presumably from one of Beethoven's many moves. And she is quite clear that when he played for her he seated himself on a chair (perhaps at a fourth piano with legs?).

There is no other contemporary account of pianos on the floor, but the image of Beethoven mutilating his instrument and contorting his body to hear music through the floorboards robustly persists. Why? Perhaps the story still circulates because of its truthiness: it seems right to think that Beethoven would take any extreme measure necessary to honor his commitment to his muse. A story that Beethoven placed a rod between his teeth and then touched it to his piano has also been widely circulated, despite a comparable lack of documentary evidence that he actually did this.[8] Both legends convey what is undoubtedly a particle of truth: Beethoven's relationship to his pianos, and to the sounds that emerged from them, was an extremely physical one, and it became more, not less, so as his hearing grew worse. While he may never have played it on the floor, Beethoven's physical interaction with the piano and the tactile experiences it had to offer are an important part of the story of his deafness.

Fortunately many instruments of Beethoven's time still survive, even if their condition is rarely ideal; a two-hundred-year-old piano that can still be played on has usually been extensively rebuilt and may not sound like it did when it was new. In recent years a wealth of modern instruments have been built to the specifications of pianos from Beethoven's time, and these probably give the best idea of what his pianos originally sounded like. The results can be heard on recordings by specialists like Malcolm Bilson, Tom Beghin, and Andrew Willis, to name but a few. Beghin has recently had two duplicates of Beethoven's Broadwood piano, which he owned during the final decade of his life, built by the Belgian maker Chris Maene; they presumably look, feel, and sound like Beethoven's did when it left the factory in England in late 1817. Thanks to these efforts Beethoven's pianistic world is coming into ever clearer focus for those who can hear and play these instruments.

Modern pianists must use caution, however. A late-eighteenth- or early-nineteenth-century piano does not look or feel like the pianos we are used to. Even the grand pianos are small and delicate-looking, with fewer keys and with frames made entirely of wood. The hammers are covered in leather.

The tones are much quieter and fade more quickly than those of today's instruments. The key-dip—the distance the keys travel to produce the notes—is much shallower, and the entire action is lighter. It seems that the pianist barely needs to touch the keys to cause them to sound. Instead of a pedal, the dampers are released by a hand stop or a knee lever, whose use is reserved for special effects. To make the instrument effective, one must play with a light, articulate touch and short phrases, delivered in a conversational or even oratorical manner: a style of playing that brings the music of the late eighteenth century to life in exciting ways.[9]

A player accustomed to bearing down to produce what modern pianists consider a solid tone may initially feel unable to control the sound of one of these older instruments. For this very reason, though, such a player would become acutely aware that the piano was not simply an extension of him- or herself.[10] Even someone intimately familiar with the classical piano repertory needs to get to know the instrument, becoming acquainted with its distinctive personality traits. This is what Beethoven had to do as well, because during his lifetime the piano was constantly changing.[11]

There was no single Beethoven piano. The pianos he played were made by various firms and were often quite different from each other. Builders were always experimenting with new designs and often built each instrument to order. Viennese pianos, and German pianos generally, were vastly different from those being manufactured at the same time in England and France. Because the English piano action led more directly to the pianos we have today, it is tempting to see the English piano as more advanced and assume that Beethoven preferred his Broadwood to contemporary Viennese pianos for that reason.[12] In reality, all designs were new and subject to constant modification. The piano itself was a relatively recent development, having surpassed the harpsichord and clavichord in popularity only in the later 1780s. To play the piano at this time meant to experiment constantly, which may help to explain why Beethoven was drawn to the instrument. The piano is also complicated. It places more moving parts between player and sound than any other instrument. When the keys are pressed, hammers rise up and bounce off the strings, while dampers simultaneously rise so the strings are free to vibrate until the keys are released. It is not uncommon for other instrumentalists to express a suspicion that pianists play by remote control, using a machine to produce tone rather than generating it themselves.

Beethoven was clearly sensitive to this possibility as well. In a letter he wrote to the piano manufacturer Andreas Streicher he made these puzzling comments: "The day before yesterday I received your fortepiano, which is really first-rate. Anyone else would wish to have it for himself. And I—though you may laugh, I would have to lie if I didn't tell you that it seems too good for me. And why? Because it takes away my freedom to create my own tone."[13]

As Tilman Skowroneck explains, what Beethoven probably meant was that the Streicher instrument, despite its beautiful sound, was problematic for playing massed sonorities and *sforzati*—sudden strong emphases on individual notes—since it did not have a backcheck: an extra rail to catch the hammers and prevent them from rebounding if they were struck too hard. The Streicher pianos sounded pretty, but if they were pushed to produce too much sound too quickly, their mechanical construction was not up to the challenge. Beethoven is known to have preferred the pianos made by Streicher's Viennese rival Anton Walter because they allowed for greater flexibility in playing the big, powerful sonic effects that abound in his early piano sonatas.[14] Though Beethoven was friendly with Streicher and his wife Nanette, it is unlikely that he had as much influence over the pianos they produced as has sometimes been suggested. Skowroneck, who has researched Beethoven's pianos extensively, describes Streicher as "an intelligent yet pronouncedly traditional man who resisted innovation when he felt it threatened the quality of the firm's work," and he rejects the idea, popularized by Tia DeNora and others, that Beethoven single-handedly reformed the nature of the piano by pushing for larger and more sonorous instruments.[15] Edwin M. Good concurs, at least as far as the instrument's range:

> Beethoven's piano music reflects the instruments of his day, and the extensions of range in it exactly parallel the extensions of range in the pianos that he—and his potential customers—possessed. I know of not one shred of evidence that Beethoven influenced any piano maker, directly or indirectly, to enlarge the range of any piano. The problem of the relations between pianists or composers and piano makers is an intricate one. . . . But Beethoven was not one of those who influenced piano makers.[16]

It is easy to imagine that today's pianos, with their louder volume, wider range, and sturdy construction, would have appealed to Beethoven had he been able to hear them. The iron frame of the modern instrument allows the strings to be stretched under enormous pressure, and the felt-covered hammers are larger and more powerful than their leather-covered predecessors. The bass strings cross above the higher ones so their sounds can reinforce each other. A nine-foot grand piano can easily fill a large hall with sound. Surely, the reasoning goes, if Beethoven had known the modern instruments, he would have preferred them to the ones at his disposal.

But what if Beethoven did not have an ideal piano sound in his head? We know that he wrote his compositions using the pens, pencils, and paper available to him. Likewise, he produced his "own tone" at the piano by playing the instruments he had on hand. The pianos of the late eighteenth and early nineteenth centuries, with their smaller wooden frames, produced a relatively small sound (to our ears) that is nevertheless rich in nuance. Hearing Beethoven's music played on them can be illuminating. His dense bass writing, which can easily sound muddy on modern pianos, comes to life in exciting ways. Technical passages can also be less challenging. The finale of the *Waldstein* Sonata, op. 53, for example, contains glissandos[17] in octaves that are virtually impossible to play with the deep key-dip that is essential to the modern piano sound; someone playing on an older instrument can simply glide over them as Beethoven intended.

As Skowroneck has carefully demonstrated, Beethoven experimented with each new instrument to find out what it could and couldn't do. What mattered to him was not the sound in the abstract but whether he could control the sound to his satisfaction. On the instruments he favored, he was able to produce a sound that was uniquely his—what he called "my own tone" in the letter to Streicher. He knew he was producing it when he liked what he heard, and at the same time he was acutely aware of the physical motions he performed to generate it because he had discovered those motions on his own. The resulting sound came into being not despite the instruments but because of them. The motions, in turn, would have stayed with him even as his hearing declined, though it is clear that he pounded on his later instruments in a way he never would have done at the height of his performing career.[18] Increasingly, the greatest challenge he faced was simply to hear.

The Erard Piano: Promise and Frustration

In 1803, shortly after the Heiligenstadt crisis, Beethoven received a piano from the French firm of Sébastien Erard. Recent research has shown that this instrument was not a gift, as was long believed; Beethoven ordered it himself, though he apparently never paid the bill.[19] The mechanics inside French pianos, and in those being built in England at the time, were different from those inside Viennese pianos. They produced a bigger sound, which would naturally be desired by a man who was aware that he was losing his hearing. Beethoven was familiar with Erard pianos because Haydn—his teacher when he first came to Vienna, with whom he remained on sometimes strained if generally friendly terms—had owned one for the previous two years. Edwin Good describes Beethoven's Erard as "a fine exemplar of an English-style grand";[20] Haydn biographer Georg August Griesinger testifies that Beethoven was initially "enchanted" with his new acquisition, regarding it as vastly superior to all Viennese instruments, which "get one into the habit of a small, weak touch."[21]

Nevertheless, Beethoven had the piano modified twice shortly after he acquired it, apparently in order to lighten the action and decrease the key-dip so it would play more like a Viennese instrument. The results seem to have been disappointing, and by 1805 his initial enthusiasm for the Erard had vanished.[22]

Like virtually all information surrounding Beethoven's preferences in pianos, this story is confusing. He seems to have wanted a more powerful instrument, but once he had one he sought to make it more like the ones he was accustomed to. In the meantime, Viennese pianos also became more powerful. Nor was this a simple contest between quieter and louder instruments. The sound of the Erard was murkier, less penetrating. The dampers were sluggish, resulting in notes that rumbled together and chords that took a long time to fade. The Viennese pianos, by comparison, had clear, articulate tones that could cut through an ensemble or an orchestra with greater precision. For someone with limited hearing, their sounds might have been easier to distinguish even if the volume was not as loud. (I am indebted to Tom Beghin for the suggestion that Viennese pianos were and remained easier for Beethoven to hear. I immediately recognized that this squared completely with Barbara's experience; she could hear simple sounds more easily than dense, complex ones.) Beethoven may very well have come to realize that, hearing-wise, the Erard was not all he had hoped it would be. In the meantime, though, he had written the Fourth Piano Concerto, op. 58, and two of his best-known piano sonatas, the *Waldstein*, op. 53, and the *Appassionata*, op. 57, with the sound of this instrument in his ears and its touch under his fingers.[23]

The *Waldstein* is so familiar that many Beethoven enthusiasts will easily understand what makes its sound distinctive. Compared to most of his earlier sonatas, it is painted with a broad brush. Large sonorous chords stretch through both hands at many points in the first movement, as they do at the opening of the Fourth Concerto. The third movement begins with the left hand playing both the bass notes and the melody, with a running accompaniment in the right hand built of slowly shifting tonic and dominant harmonies. The lingering sonority of this music depends on something modern pianists take for granted but that was new to Beethoven: the Erard had a pedal to lift the dampers. This was easier to use than the hand- and knee-operated devices Beethoven was accustomed to and more suited to the repeated applications that Beethoven indicates — for the first time — in this music.[24] If Beethoven's pedal markings are followed precisely, the bass notes continue to resonate and the chords outlined by the right hand blend delicately together, but the sounds of the Erard decayed quickly enough that the harmonies would not clash uncomfortably, as can easily happen on modern pianos.[25] This was also the first piano Beethoven owned with an *una corda* pedal: the "soft pedal" on modern instruments, in the early nineteenth century it literally reduced the sound to a single string per note. Beethoven called on this effect to produce haunting sonorities throughout the second movement of the Fourth Concerto.[26] These examples confirm that Beethoven wrote music for the instruments he had, not for imagined instruments he hoped would come to be.

Soon after Beethoven acquired his Erard, Viennese piano makers like Streicher began to make larger and more sonorous instruments. Beethoven's piano music after about 1805 often contains characteristics, such as rapid fingerwork and repeated notes, that suggest he had returned to the Viennese instruments and away from the heavier French action, even though the Erard remained in his possession until 1818.[27] At the same time, Beethoven's hearing loss meant that he gave fewer public performances, and he may have begun to abuse the instruments at his disposal, breaking strings and necessitating frequent repairs.[28] He was becoming more interested in hearing his pianos than he was in maintaining them. It was probably in late 1811 that he wrote on the opening page of what is now known as the "Petter" sketchbook that putting cotton in his ears at the piano freed his hearing from "the disagreeable noise." In all likelihood he hit upon this solution while writing down the ideas at the beginning of the sketchbook, many of which do not seem to have made it into any of his finished works. He was clearly experimenting, and either because he was using a particularly loud piano or because his sensitivity to loudness had become increasingly bothersome, he improvised a solution that may have had ominous consequences. The stories of two musicians who dealt with hearing-loss issues similar to Beethoven's can help us understand how his instincts might have led him astray at this crucial juncture in his life.

Cotton in the Ears

Zachary Ridgway is one of the most brilliant students I have taught since I first stepped in front of a college classroom forty years ago. I had the good fortune of working with him both as an undergraduate and as a master's student at Baylor, and I served on his thesis committee and heard him perform several recitals. I did not learn until a few years later that while he was completing his master's degree he experienced significant inverse-spectrum hearing loss—an unusual hearing impairment that begins with the lowest notes rather than with the highest ones—that nearly derailed his career. "I began having persistent problems with my right ear," he later wrote, "a horrible excess of sound in certain pitch ranges. I could not listen to music on headphones, since to make the music audible in my left ear was to make it unbearable in my right; I could not practice at all without earplugs. To be in the same room as a clarinet or flute, to be in the same building as an organ—unthinkable!"[29]

Zachary had experienced an asymptomatic inner ear infection that affected his perception of low pitches. His auditory cortex was compensating by registering higher pitches as uncomfortably loud. This was loudness recruitment, which Beethoven had experienced two centuries earlier, and the prognosis was not any more promising. A specialist explained to Zachary "that the loudness recruitment may or may not begin gradually to correct itself, and that there was really nothing to do about this. . . . A second opinion and many articles on the subject confirmed this grim prognostication." It sounded, Zachary said, "like a certain pitch range was taking place in a boomy stairwell. And the only way to mute that was by popping in the earplugs."[30]

Zachary was lucky; his recruitment eventually did correct itself, and he now hears well enough to be pursuing a doctorate in piano. The turning point, appropriately enough, was an invitation to perform Beethoven's *Emperor* Concerto at one of the colleges where he was teaching. He forced himself to practice and to sit through the rehearsals and performance, putting in the earplugs only when the sound became unbearable. It finally dawned on him that the earplugs were making things worse, because "a component of the problem was a lack of auditory cortex stimulus in a given range . . . and I was further reducing stimulus with the earplugs." Adding more sound, particularly in the pitch range where the problem was occurring, was deeply uncomfortable, but he forced himself to do it and eventually things began to improve.[31] This was because the problem was not really in his ear; it was his brain, which, by compensating for the lack of input, was making his hearing progressively worse.

⁂

Doris DeLoach has taught oboe at Baylor for more than forty years. She has been especially sensitive to loud, high-pitched sounds her entire life: a possibly hereditary condition known as hyperacusis. In 1992 she was rehearsing for a performance of Tchaikovsky's Fifth Symphony with the Waco Symphony Orchestra when, in her words, "it felt like something in my head exploded." She felt extreme physical pain, and remaining in the rehearsal was unbearable. The next morning her ears felt clogged, but rather than having hearing loss, she found that even everyday sounds, like running bathwater, were uncomfortably loud.

She forced herself to play in the performance, bought a pair of earplugs, and continued to teach. For the next six months, though, she was constantly miserable. In her quest for a solution she finally connected with a doctor in Oregon who recommended that she listen to pink noise—a steady sound that resembles that of a waterfall—over headphones every day for as long and at as loud a volume as she could tolerate. She did this constantly for another six months and at irregular intervals for several more years. The doctor also told her not to wear earplugs, as they were only making the problem worse. Instead she fixed her hearing, paradoxically, by bombarding her ears with sound. Doris's hearing is now as good as it was before the incident in 1992, although she still has to be careful to avoid loud sounds as much as possible.

⁎

We have already seen that Beethoven's hearing was relatively stable for most of the first decade of the nineteenth century but went into rapid decline shortly afterward. He was still suffering from loudness recruitment in May 1809; the sounds of Napoleon's bombardment of Vienna were nearly unbearable for him. The previous December, though, he had been able to tolerate performing his Fourth Piano Concerto and Choral Fantasy with an orchestra. It is not exactly clear when things started to get worse and when he started to plug his ears, but it is likely that when he did so it had the opposite effect of what he had hoped. While putting cotton in his ears may have freed him from disagreeable noise while he was playing, it made him work even harder to hear the sounds he knew were there, producing further distortion and progressively damaging the connection between his ears, his auditory nerves, and the hearing cortex in his brain. While this, like so much else pertaining to

Beethoven's hearing loss, must remain only speculation, the final decline of his hearing may thus have become inevitable, brought on by his own actions.[32]

Hearing Machines

At the same time, Beethoven took other steps that proved more beneficial. While he was working in the Petter sketchbook, he developed a close friendship with Johann Nepomuk Mälzel, whose ear trumpets, as we saw in chapter 1, form an important part of the legend of Beethoven's deafness. Mälzel, who was a relentless self-promoter but must also have been something of a mechanical genius, constructed an artificial orchestra, known as the panharmonicon, for which he was able to induce Beethoven to compose *Wellington's Victory*, a largescale musical depiction of the Battle of Victoria. He is also remembered for perfecting the metronome, although he is no longer considered its inventor; that distinction rightly belongs to Dietrich Nikolaus Winkel. It is typical of Mälzel's relationship with Beethoven that he repeatedly urged the composer to supply metronome markings for his compositions; these controversial markings probably did more to promote Mälzel and his machine than they did to enlighten us about Beethoven's music.[33] Indeed, as Beverly Jerold points out, the question of how a composer with limited hearing would supply metronome markings based largely on input from his eyes is one that deserves much further exploration.[34]

Thayer learned about Mälzel's activities in Vienna years later from Carl Stein (1797–1863), son of the Viennese piano manufacturer Matthäus Andreas Stein (1776–1842), in whose factory Mälzel set up his workshop around 1809. According to Stein, Beethoven visited Mälzel frequently, the two became close friends, and Mälzel began, probably in 1812, to build mechanical hearing aids for Beethoven.[35]

Mälzel's inventions are often called ear trumpets, a distinctly English term that Beethoven and his German-speaking contemporaries never used; the standard German word is *Hörrohr*, or hearing tube.[36] The devices themselves, though, had first become commercially available in late-eighteenth-century England, so use of the English term is appropriate.[37] Ear trumpets were inspired by the megaphones that sea captains, in particular, used to project their voices at a distance; they simply served the opposite purpose, that of collecting sound and directing it into the ear.[38] They came in a wide variety of shapes and sizes, but they all operated by reversing the normal decay of sound over distance. As sound entered the trumpet, it was concentrated into a progressively smaller space until it finally arrived at the ear, usually through a hole in a small end piece. In some cases a resonating chamber also served to collect the sound, selectively amplifying those pitches that vibrated freely within it. By concentrating the pitches characteristic of human speech, this chamber could make it much easier for the user to understand voices and participate in conversation.[39] Two of the surviving ear trumpets made by Mälzel for Beethoven have resonating chambers; three do not.[40]

The use of an ear trumpet in a social setting is intriguingly described by Nathaniel Hawthorne. He based his account on his observation of the English writer Harriet Martineau (1802–76), who had suffered profound hearing loss as a child.

All the while she talks she moves the bowl of her ear-trumpet from one auditor to another, so that it becomes quite an organ of intelligence and sympathy between her and yourself. The ear-trumpet seems a sensible part of her,

like the antennae of some insects. If you have any little re-
mark to make, you drop it in; and she helps you to make
remarks by this delicate little appeal of the trumpet, as she
slightly directs it towards you, and if you have nothing to
say, the appeal is not strong enough to embarrass you.[41]

Hawthorne's description is intriguing because it suggests
both that Martineau used this device quite successfully and
that others were willing to see it as a sense organ in its own
right: an extension of her ear that allowed her to take the lead
in group conversations, which is precisely where people with
hearing loss often feel most helpless. Martineau herself believed that her ear trumpet imparted a "new feeling . . . of ease
and privacy in conversing with a deaf person. . . . I can hardly
imagine fuller revelations to be made in household intercourse
than my trumpet brought to me."[42]

The devices Mälzel built for Beethoven were similar to
those that had been available in England for several decades,
as the worldly Mälzel was no doubt aware. His influence may
also have reached back to England: the so-called Martineau
hearing horn, later marketed by S. Maw and Son, shows the
same distinctive "salt-shaker" design as one of Mälzel's models,
with a grill over the resonating chamber, albeit one that sits inside the chamber rather than on top of it.[43] The so-called banjo
trumpet, introduced in England around 1860, used a parabolic
bucket as a resonator; it also resembles one of Mälzel's designs,
although Mälzel's has a simple conical bucket with a flat base.[44]
Mälzel's trumpets were made of brass, while those made in England were originally made of tin; when somebody was said to
have a "tin ear," it meant they were using one.[45]

Mälzel's work on these devices was closely associated with
his and Beethoven's collaboration on *Wellington's Victory*. Beethoven allowed Mälzel to plan the structure of this piece,

granting him a kind of creative input he never gave to anybody else.[46] When, again at Mälzel's behest, Beethoven later rescored it for full orchestra and then pocketed the considerable earnings from the series of triumphant performances that followed, there was a falling out between the two that led to an extended, and ultimately unresolved, court case. In the legal deposition he filed during that case in July 1814, Beethoven stated that Mälzel had promised him "hearing machines" (*gehör Maschinen*) in return for writing the piece. To support his claim that this was inadequate compensation, Beethoven stated that the machines had been "insufficiently useful for me." Earlier that year, though, when he thought the quarrel with Mälzel was about to be patched up, Beethoven had asked his friend Nikolaus Zmeskall to "bring the hearing machines back with you, since the whole thing [presumably the quarrel with Mälzel] is no longer necessary."[47] Beethoven must have given Mälzel's inventions to Zmeskall for safekeeping, and now he wanted them back.[48]

Beethoven's use of terminology is intriguing. When *Wellington's Victory* was published in 1816 (unusually, for the time, in score), Beethoven included a set of instructions indicating that "cannon machines," consisting of pairs of large bass drums, should be placed on each side of the orchestra, and that machines "similar to those used in theaters to produce thunderclaps" should simulate the sound of small arms fire.[49] These arrangements were probably worked out at the first performance in collaboration with Mälzel, whose "hearing machines" can thus be seen as part of the same project: the cannon machines in the orchestra produced loud noises; the hearing machines used by Beethoven made it possible for him to hear them. Mälzel could thus claim credit for using machines both to produce unusual sounds and to help an increasingly deaf composer hear his own music. In 1814 Beethoven wrote about this in his diary. The original text of that diary has unfortunately been lost, but it is clear from the surviving copies that he speculated on the possibility of an "ear machine" with star-shaped holes at the opening that would convey sound to his ear in a way that would allow him to hear things from all directions. This reads like a description of Mälzel's salt-shaker trumpet or of the later Martineau horn. In an entry from the next year Beethoven endorsed Mälzel's designs, while also stating that there was another unnamed manufacturer whose products he preferred.[50] This suggests that he might have used a wider range of them than is commonly recognized.

In the autumn of 1817, Beethoven must have borrowed a hearing aid from the piano manufacturer Nanette Streicher, since he told her in a letter that he was returning it and asked her to send it back the next day.[51] This time, though, he used the word *Sprachrohr*, which literally means "speaking tube." He may well have been referring to a different device, or a different design, from the ones built by Mälzel, which were by then several years old. But he may also still have been stinging from comments published the previous year by the critic Gottfried Weber, who denounced what he saw as the shallow scene-painting in *Wellington's Victory*.[52] If his goal was to make his music sound like real life, Weber wrote, "Mr. van Beethoven would actually be more in the wrong for not having set up moaning machines (as a substitute for actual death moans) instead of painting the moans of the dying very strikingly and truly movingly with notes, as he did—whizzing machines for the whizzing of the large and small bullets, clanking machines for the clanking of bayonets, swords and ramrods, cursing machines, neighing machines, etc."[53] Beethoven seems never to have referred to his ear trumpets as "hearing machines" again.[54]

In 1820, however, Beethoven was still discussing the use of Mälzel's ear trumpets with his friends.[55] August von Kloeber, who must have visited him later that same year, reported that Beethoven still used an ear trumpet to understand speech.[56] Louis Schlösser—not the most reliable of sources—described Beethoven using an ear trumpet as late as 1823.[57] It is hard to imagine he would have continued using them for this long if they had not helped him to hear better. Tests done on a variety of ear trumpets under controlled conditions at the Central Institute for the Deaf in St. Louis, Missouri, suggest that they could produce an audible gain of more than twenty decibels and that this improvement was often concentrated in specific pitch ranges, usually corresponding to normal speech.[58] By comparison, cupping one's hand over the ear produces a gain of only three to ten decibels.[59] Because the decibel scale is logarithmic, this is a greater difference than the simple numbers might suggest, even though those numbers mirror perceived differences in loudness.

I had the opportunity to put these findings to the test when the staff of the Beethoven-Haus in Bonn let me try out two exact replicas of the Mälzel ear trumpets in their possession. The results were stunning. They delivered a sound quality, clarity, and degree of amplification that I had not expected to encounter with preelectronic equipment. The main difficulty with their use is logistic: they have to be held constantly in position.

The large horn, which I tried first, is easy to cradle in a single hand and has a relatively big opening that nevertheless fits easily into the ear. I immediately noticed that I was hearing environmental sounds at significant amplification, with no distraction from internal sounds such as one might hear with a seashell or other closed container. The sound of the librarian turning pages on the other side of the room registered with eerie clarity. When she spoke to me from a distance of about ten feet, she sounded much louder through the ear trumpet and there was virtually no metallic distortion, no "tinny" quality to her voice. Nor was it necessary to have her speak directly into the trumpet, although when she did so, at low volume, every nuance of her speech came through clearly.

Listening to music with the large horn was also a very satisfactory experience. A recording of a piano played at low volume came through with great clarity; it gained presence and the sound had considerable depth. There was a tiny amount of metallic ringing in the higher notes, but this helped them to stand out clearly.

The ear trumpet with a conical resonator was harder to use, since it was much heavier. The sounds I heard through it, though, were several notches louder than those from the simple horn, albeit with some muddiness in fuller-sounding passages. Paradoxically, contrapuntal voices in music stood out with great clarity, both in piano music and in a recording of a string

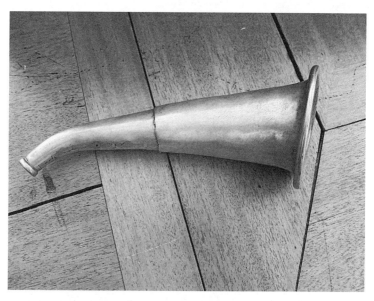

FIGURE 5. The replica of the "large horn" ear trumpet
that I tested at the Beethoven-Haus in Bonn

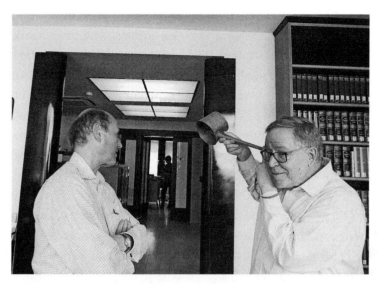

FIGURE 6. The author (right) converses with Beethoven-Haus curator Dr. Michael Ladenburger using a replica of the ear trumpet with conical resonator and headband

quartet. High notes were almost painfully loud, even though the music was playing at low volume.

This was a mind-bending experience for me as a Beethoven scholar and a lifelong devotee of his music. I was sitting in the building next to Beethoven's birthplace and hearing with his "ears." Of course I did not have his hearing loss to contend with, but I had the memory of using the pocket talker to communicate with Barbara, which was in some ways similar. Both were awkward to use; you couldn't just leave them in place and forget they were there. It has been noted that two of the Mälzel ear trumpets have headbands attached, and the duplicate of the one with the resonator that I tried had one as well. It soon became clear, though, that Beethoven could not have used it to free up his hands, as has sometimes been suggested. The ear trumpet was too heavy and awkward, and at least one hand was needed to hold it at all times. Two were preferable; I put it in my right ear and used my left hand to make sure it stayed there, while using the right to support it and point it at the sound source. Beethoven could not have played the piano while using it, so it probably did not play a direct role in his composing activity, but he could easily have listened to music by others and might have guided conversations in the manner described by Martineau.

My anecdotal experience suggests that the quality of sound Beethoven received from his ear trumpets was good and relatively free of distortion, with particular emphasis in the high range, where he needed it most. Contrary to what is often suggested, these were clearly superb hearing aids, crafted specifically for Beethoven by a man of great skill and ingenuity. And beginning in 1820, Beethoven had help from yet another novel invention.

The Broadwood and the Resonator

Beethoven received a piano from the English manufacturer Thomas Broadwood in 1818 (it was actually sent at the end of the previous year). This instrument has become an important part of the legend surrounding the composer and his music. For many years it was assumed that Beethoven immediately preferred this piano, with its bigger sound and heavier action, to the Viennese instruments of his time. As a result, the names Broadwood and Beethoven are often closely linked: the former for promoting a type of instrument from which the modern piano action eventually developed; the latter for embracing this instrument and, by implication, the future. The fact that Beethoven was working at the time on the *Hammerklavier* Sonata, op. 106—one of the largest and most uncompromising pieces in the keyboard literature—has only reinforced these impressions. However, three of its four movements were already nearly completed by the time the Broadwood arrived in Vienna.

The long-prevailing view of the Broadwood was called into question in 1988 with the publication of William S. Newman's book *Beethoven on Beethoven: Playing His Piano Music His Way.* Newman argued that "the three pianos chiefly identified with Beethoven today (the Érard, the Broadwood, and the Graf) have been highlighted well beyond their musical value to him, to the extent of obscuring quite different preferences that he himself revealed in one way or another." The reality, Newman insisted, is that Beethoven continued to prefer Viennese pianos until the end of his life.[60]

More recently Tilman Skowroneck has in turn called Newman's view into question: "The fact that Beethoven was conflicted about almost everything and everyone during his last decade should alert us to the possibility that even his relationship to the Broadwood may have been erratic to some degree."[61] Skowroneck goes on to point out that Beethoven carried the instrument to his summer quarters and back and used it heavily for years, doubtless neglecting its tuning and proper maintenance.[62] Regardless of Beethoven's stated preferences, the Broadwood evidently played an important role in his life and work. Beginning with the last movement of the *Hammerklavier*, he adjusted the compass of his keyboard works so they did not go above C7, which was the highest note available on the Broadwood; most Viennese instruments of the time extended to the F above it.[63]

It is easy to understand why Beethoven would have been both pleased and dissatisfied with the Broadwood. On a recent visit to Belgium I had the opportunity to hear Tom Beghin perform the last three Beethoven piano sonatas in Ghent on one of the two Broadwood replicas built by Chris Maene, and to play it myself. The following day I visited Maene's workshop in Ruiselede, where I played the other one. Both are modeled on the Broadwood on display at the Beethoven-Haus, which was built in 1817—the same year as Beethoven's, to which it is virtually identical. Though each has its own personality, both are likely to strike modern listeners as having a larger sound than that of Viennese pianos of Beethoven's time. As Beghin pointed out, though, this doesn't mean that they were easier for Beethoven to hear.[64] Like that of the Erard, their sound is rich and a bit murky, and lacks the clear, bell-like treble of the instruments to which he was accustomed. If Beethoven hoped to hear better with the Broadwood, he was probably disappointed.

The tactile experience of the instrument, though, must have appealed to him powerfully in a variety of ways. The keys are deep and "spongy," requiring and rewarding more finger action than is needed for Viennese pianos. The frame of the instrument vibrates with great uniformity, since unlike those of Viennese instruments, it is directly connected to the sound board, giving the player a powerful physical connection with the sounds being produced.[65] That Beethoven made such a connection is evident at many points in the last three sonatas—much more so than in the finale of the *Hammerklavier*, which in Beghin's view fails to celebrate fully the unique qualities of the new instrument, even though it fits the Broadwood's six-octave range and was clearly written with it in mind.[66] Missing from that work are passages like mm. 105ff. from the last movement of the next sonata, Opus 109 in E major (the second half of Variation IV), in which a series of rocking chords relentlessly crescendos, decked out with accents and sforzandos, only to give way to the cascading arabesques in contrary motion with which the variation concludes (example 5.1). When I played this passage on Maene's Broadwood replicas, the music pulsed and throbbed beneath my fingers in a way I have never

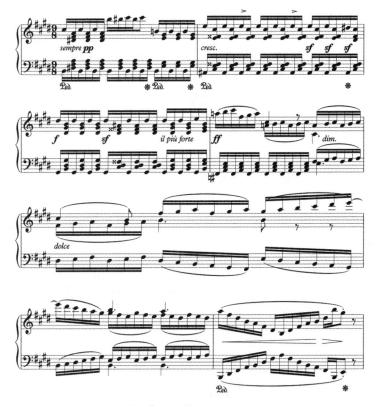

EXAMPLE 5.1. Beethoven, Piano Sonata no. 30 in E major,
op. 109, 3rd movement, mm. 106–112 (second half of Variation
IV, modified to show only the second ending)

felt on a modern piano, and which Beethoven would certainly
not have expected from the Viennese instruments to which he
was accustomed. In the program notes for his recently released
recording of the last three Beethoven sonatas on the Maene
Broadwood, Tom Beghin explains the effect this way:

> Because of their precise action and articulatory focus, Vi-
> ennese pianos call for a clear differentiation between disso-
> nance and consonance—the former to be played louder, the

latter softer (as a resolution of the former). But at the outset of the fourth variation, gorgeous pairs of appoggiatura and resolution elide with one another, almost to the point of the one negating the harmonic function of the other. This is a rather drastic shift in harmonic thinking, and Beethoven's explorations must have been based on touch rather than sound: every tone or key on an English-action piano requires an individual finger stroke, while a Viennese-action piano allows for the second of a slurred two-note pair to be hung onto the previous one, requiring only a gentle, caressing stroke of the resolving finger. Without physical clarity of good (or strong) versus bad (or weak), the duality easily reverses to bad versus good. What starts mattering more, then, is the sine wave of the oscillation itself: the up and down of it (or, as the case may be, the down and up). In this variation, Beethoven taps into the accumulating energy of a relentless play of back-and-forth vibration, first cautiously and softly, then with ever-increased vigor and obsession.[67]

I then tried the repeated G major chords toward the end of the Sonata in A-flat Major, op. 110, which I suggested in chapter 1 show Beethoven striving toward the threshold of audibility. Here again the vibration of the instrument quickly became palpable—all the more so due to the *una corda* marking, directing the performer to use the left, or "soft," pedal. On the Broadwood this literally results in only one string being struck by each hammer, enforcing their tendency to resonate together. Beethoven's piano was not tuned the way modern pianos are, in equal temperament, which makes all half steps identical. Instead there were subtle but significant differences between one key and another, and G major chords would have resounded strongly due to the purity of the intervals they contained.[68] Thus it is highly significant that Beethoven wrote this passage in G rather than in the tonic of A-flat. In order to get as close as possible to Beethoven's experience, I put on noise-blocking earmuffs so what I actually heard was reduced to a minimum. By the time I played the final chord, the entire instrument was resonating beneath my hands in a way I could feel more than hear, and with the damper pedal held down as Beethoven indicated it continued to do so throughout the two measures that followed, even though I was playing only single notes with a rapid diminuendo. Regardless of how much Beethoven could hear, he must have found playing this passage deeply satisfying.

He must have also yearned to hear better, though, because within two years of receiving the Broadwood the conversation books show that he was actively planning a new device that could be placed over the piano and would amplify its sound by deflecting it back toward the player.[69] This was the resonator that was mentioned by several visitors in the 1820s, for which the one made by Graf in 1826 was intended as a substitute. Confusingly, Beethoven and his friends began referring to it as a "hearing machine," the same term he had stopped using for his ear trumpets. It was apparently inspired by an invention of Dr. Sigmund Wolfsohn, a prolific creator of medical appliances. Wolfsohn falsely claimed, in the Wiener *Conversationsblatt* of February 29, 1820, that Beethoven had benefited from a hearing aid of his design, "a clever apparatus in the form of a flat-pressed diadem, which is covered by a toupee, [and] can be worn undetected." A rebuttal appeared on March 9, clarifying that "Herr van Beethoven indeed inspected that machine, but has never made use of it."[70] Nevertheless, Beethoven continued to converse with Wolfsohn about a wooden device consisting of a box and tubes to go into the ears.[71] (Remember that the German word *Rohr*, or tube, was used by Beethoven for the ear trumpets manufactured by Mälzel.)

Then, in mid-March, Beethoven and Matthäus Andreas Stein

began to discuss building an amplifier with two horns (*zwey Horn*) directed at Beethoven's ears. A flurry of conversations quickly followed, showing a lively interest on both Stein's and Beethoven's part in the design of the new resonator. Stein proposed building an arch over the piano and offered to make a prototype from cardboard, then to borrow the piano so he could build one from wood in his shop.[72]

On April 4, Beethoven was still musing to himself about a different idea: "*Using a type of mechanical device, couldn't a couple of hearing devices be made, through which the necessary movement of air* be restored for the sound for the ear?"[73] Sixteen days later, though, his frequent factotum Franz Oliva informed him,

> I think that one should not talk any longer, but instead should begin to experiment, in order to make progress. With wood, there is no difference in the price; but Herr Stein thinks that *brass* would be better than wood, also because of the flexibility of brass, because the machine must be round, and this round shape is difficult to accomplish with wood. Stein knows a worker who is skillful and reasonably-priced, [and] he will speak with him.[74]

Stein ultimately seems to have persuaded Beethoven to let him build the proposed arch from "a newly invented kind of brass, called sheet-zinc."[75]

By late June, Stein was apparently far enough along to experiment with attaching cardboard tubes to the device in his workshop, and he asked to borrow one of Mälzel's ear trumpets so he could see how it might be incorporated.[76] Beethoven probably received the piano back on or around September 7,[77] and Stein promised to return "the other machines"—presumably ear trumpets he had borrowed—in a few days, as they were not yet ready.[78] This suggests that he was still working on a way to attach them to the resonator so Beethoven could use them while keeping his hands free. None of the surviving descriptions, though, mentions the use of ear trumpets in connection with the finished device, so it is likely Beethoven and Stein decided this was unworkable or unnecessary.

How exactly did Stein's resonator work, and how much benefit did Beethoven receive from it? As with so much else pertaining to Beethoven's deafness, the evidence is confusing. There is an intriguing commentary by August von Kloeber, who painted a portrait of Beethoven and his nephew that must date from no earlier than 1820, because when he visited the composer the Broadwood piano was equipped with the now-completed resonator.[79] Kloeber described Beethoven instructing his nephew Karl, who was seated at the piano with the resonator in place; Kloeber called it a "large cupola of sheet metal." "Beethoven now sat down. . . . The instrument stood approximately four to five paces behind him, and Beethoven, despite his deafness, corrected every mistake that the young man made."[80] If we take this literally, Karl must have been in the direct path of the reflected sound. Beethoven, however, was able to correct Karl's mistakes even though he was facing away from the instrument. Unless Kloeber was misremembering—which is entirely possible given the fact that his account was written over four decades later—Beethoven heard Karl's playing well enough to correct his mistakes without watching his fingers. Kloeber also stated that Beethoven had an ear trumpet (*Rohr*) on hand and could not understand speech without it, unless Karl shouted directly into his ear. For the reasons described earlier in this chapter, I find it unlikely that Beethoven ever used an ear trumpet while playing. It is quite possible, though, that Beethoven also used the ear trumpet while Karl played, pointing it back toward the piano so it would collect the sound projected toward him by the cupola. Just as when he had written to Wegeler twenty years earlier, his perception of music must have been much better than his perception of speech, and Stein's sheet-metal cupola probably deserves a good deal of the credit.

All of these stories probably need to be viewed with a healthy skepticism. In a fascinating article, K. M. Knittel has shown that virtually all who visited Beethoven late in life had a personal agenda, and their accounts are often fictionalized so as to aggrandize themselves. Describing Beethoven accurately was often the least of their concerns.[81] Kloeber was clearly wrong about either the year in which he met Beethoven or about the piano he had at the time, so there is good reason to take the rest of his account with a grain of salt. Two further testimonials complicate the story even further. Friedrich Wieck heard Beethoven improvise in 1823 and attested both to the high quality of his playing and to his use of a "hearing machine" which he attached to the sound board of the piano.[82] No other witness speaks of a direct connection with the sound board. Johann Andreas Stumpff, who heard Beethoven play in 1824, spoke of "a large half angle of sound board wood, which was closed off at both ends and rose over the keys of the piano, from the bass to the treble, so that the player's head was covered by the height of the half circle."[83] It is possible that Stumpff was describing a later version of Stein's resonator, in which the metal had been replaced by wood. This in turn might have served as a model for the resonator built by Graf, which Samuel Heinrich Spiker, who visited Beethoven in 1826, described as "a kind of sound container, beneath which he sat when he played, and which was designed to capture the sound and concentrate it around him."[84]

While we may never know exactly what Beethoven's resonator looked like, I was fortunate enough to be present at an attempt to reconstruct it (fig. 7). At Chris Maene's workshop in

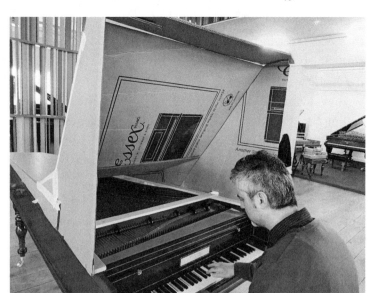

FIGURE 7. Tom Beghin plays one of the Maene
Broadwoods with the square cardboard resonator.

Ruiselede, the acoustician Thomas Wulfrank had built two pro-
totypes, both from cardboard, as we know Stein initially did as
well, although Wulfrank also drew on Gerhard von Breuning's
description of the device Beethoven later had constructed for
his Graf piano. One of Wulfrank's models was rounded, con-
cave, and tapered toward the back. The other was a square box
that was very high over the keys, with a forward reflector at
a sharper than 45-degree angle and a very low cover for the
back part of the instrument. Both of these were designed to
replace the piano's normal lid, which deflects sound off to the
side, and direct it toward the player instead. Tom Beghin and
I each played passages from opp. 109 and 110 with both models in place, and we agreed that the square model was superior,
even though the rounded model corresponded more clearly
to the contemporary descriptions of the one built by Stein.

It produced a full sound with little distortion—much louder than that of the instrument by itself, but not uncomfortable for someone used to playing a modern grand. It was easy to imagine Beethoven sitting where we did, completely surrounded by the tangible vibrations that he coaxed from the instrument, feeling them even more strongly with the resonator in place. Indeed, as I played the repeated G major chords from Opus 110 with the earmuffs and the resonator, I must have come very close to Beethoven's own experience. A small amount of sound was still audible, but it was nearly overwhelmed by the sheer physicality of the vibrations coming from the instrument and filling up the enclosed space around it.

Those listening to the piano, on the other hand—it was on a small stage in front of several rows of auditorium seats—heard the amplified sound as full and rounded, lending credence to Kloeber's account of Beethoven correcting Karl's mistakes in 1820 with his back to the instrument. There would have been plenty of sound for him to hear, more than any piano up to that point had ever produced.[85]

How might all of this have played out in Beethoven's creative life? The last movement of opus 109 offers some interesting clues. Work on this sonata seems to have begun in March 1820 and to have been complete by the end of September. Beethoven most likely finished the first movement in March or April but did little work on the sonata for the next few months, then scrambled to complete it by late September. His work on the last movement can be found in two sources: the Artaria 195 sketchbook edited and transcribed by William Kinderman and one bifolium, known as A47, from a Concept Draft, or preliminary version of the entire sonata. This fragment contains Variations 2 and 3 from the last movement, and it was apparently discarded because Beethoven decided at the last minute to make a substantial change to the first of these.[86] With these facts as background, we can imagine Beethoven at work:

I haven't looked at this sonata for a while. Earlier in the summer I sketched out a series of variations, but there were too many of them and some of them didn't seem to be going anywhere. Here it is early September and I need to figure out which ones will really work musically. Now that I have the Broadwood back, why don't I try them out using that resonator that Stein built? Maybe I'll even come up with some new ideas.

(Some experimentation follows.)

What a difference! I already liked the feel of that instrument, but with that box for the sound to knock around in, repeated chords have a punch I would never have expected. That gives me a whole new sense of how these variations might go.

(Begins writing out the concept draft of the third movement.)

It's a good thing I got that instrument back! That second variation I just came up with [mm. 41–48 and 57–64 of the finished sonata, which appear on their own in A47] never would have occurred to me otherwise. And just starting with simple repeated chords in the left hand—no need to even write those down. Switching to those sixteenth-note chords alternating between the hands, though—it's a good thing I put down a little bit more there, since that effect was so stunning I want to make sure I can remember it.

(Writes out two more variations.)

That third variation is going to surprise some people. But the fourth one—thank goodness for that piano again! Such simple repeated chords in the second half, but with those shifting accents and crescendos they came alive as I never would have imagined. Now I'm wondering, though: maybe there's too much of that kind of thing in this movement. That fourth variation worked because I started with something more subtle and didn't go for the big effect until the second half. Maybe I could do something similar in the second one.

(Sets aside the bifolium containing Variations 2 and 3.)

That first idea I had for how to start the second variation just might work after all. Let me look back in those sketches. Ah yes, here it is [fig. 8]! I'll need to tinker with the pitches a bit, but I think it needs something else too: something to make it flow more smoothly. In fact, look at that! Those notes on the page do flow. It's almost too bad the engraver will make them all line up. I like what I'm seeing here better. Now here's a challenge; how can I write this out so it's clear I don't want the hands to play at the same time?

(Starts writing Variation 2 again, making it clear that the notes should not align but should alternate in a regular pattern between the two hands.)

Yes, I like that. Isn't that something? The piano helped me out, but so did my messy first draft where I didn't bother to line the hands up properly. Well, I'll take my ideas wherever I can get them!

I hope I can be excused for the indulgence of placing myself inside Beethoven's head. I think it is possible he had the kind of experiences I imagine, having had most of them myself while playing passages from Opus 109 on the Maene Broadwoods, with and without the resonator in place. Beethoven probably received his Broadwood back from Stein with the resonator in early September, when he was still at Mödling. Artaria 195, the sketchbook he had been using, contains no sketches for Variation 4 or for the second part of either half of Variation 2,[87] so

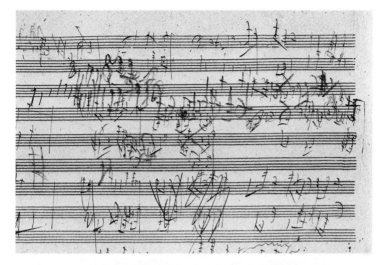

FIGURE 8. Page 56 of Beethoven's sketchbook Artaria 195. Source:
William Kinderman, ed., *Artaria 195: Beethoven's Sketchbook
for the "Missa Solemnis" and the Piano Sonata in E Major, Opus
109*, vol. 2 (Urbana: University of Illinois Press, 2003).

these were clearly among the last things he wrote before the sonata was completed, probably by the end of the month.[88] Both
variations bring out the vibrational qualities of the instrument
to particularly good effect—the continuing resolution of one
dissonance into another that Tom Beghin noted in the fourth
variation is already present in the second—and their physical effect would have been even more evident with the resonator. The sketches on page 56 of Artaria 195 resemble what
eventually became the beginning of Variation 2, which come
second in what appears to have been a projected set of nine
variations.[89] Beethoven originally conceived this passage as a
series of eighth notes, each followed by a sixteenth note and a
sixteenth-note rest. The way he wrote it, though—typically for
a preliminary sketch—shows little concern for alignment between the hands; in fact, the hands appear to alternate in quick

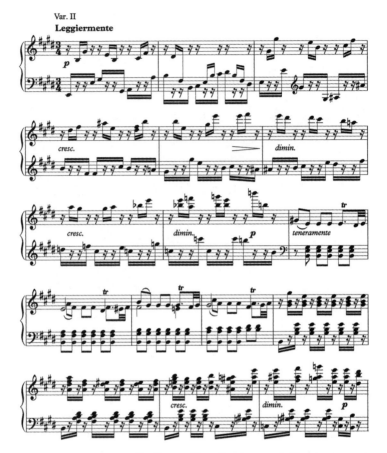

EXAMPLE 5.2. Beethoven, Piano Sonata no. 30 in E major,
op. 109, 3rd movement, mm. 33–48 (first half of Variation II)

succession. If he went back to this sketch to complete Variation 2 after removing the original version of it from A47, he
might have let his eyes take the lead in transforming this first
draft into the tripping rhythmic exchange between the hands
that appears in the finished sonata (example 5.2).

Here, then, is an example of Beethoven moving back and
forth between his sketchbook and the keyboard to create this

intriguing double variation, each section of which reflects a different kind of physical interaction with the materials at hand. This richly imagined scene suggests that while we should perhaps not take the many stories about Beethoven's ear trumpets and resonators too literally, neither should we ignore these artifacts and their significance. The conversation books, the letters, and the *Tagebuch* make it clear just how important they were to Beethoven. It is fair to say that to the fullest extent possible, he used existing technology to his benefit. It is likely that, just as it did with Barbara two centuries later, this technology both surprised and disappointed him, often at one and the same time.

The next chapter will begin with a quick look at some recent research into how the sense of hearing operates, in order to understand better how people like Beethoven and Barbara can reach beyond their ears to compensate for its loss.

* 6 *
Ears, Eyes, and Mind

"Someone's crying, Lord, kumbayah." From our lips to God's ears. The common understanding of sound is that it is "out there" and that the job of our sense of hearing is to pick it up and convey it to our brain. Speech, music, insect sounds: they're all information that simply needs to register in order to be understood.

On second thought, common sense tells us otherwise. People hear things differently. A very small percentage of people—and a higher percentage of musicians—have perfect pitch, which allows them to distinguish between C and C# the same way others tell red from green. Most of us have no idea what it would be like to be able to do this. Speakers of tonal languages, like Mandarin Chinese, can easily hear minor differences of pitch inflection that give completely different meanings to words that sound nearly identical to everybody else. The word *ma*, for example, can mean either horse or mother, and it has two other meanings as well, since Mandarin has four distinct pronunciation tones that affect the way every vowel sound is heard and understood. Other languages are even richer: Cantonese has seven tones; standard Vietnamese has six. People familiar with particular traditions of African drumming can tell the difference between rhythms that the rest of us find indistinguish-able. And the list goes on.

It is the same with the other senses. A fascinating episode of *Radiolab* that aired in 2012 investigated the perception of color and came to some surprising conclusions. William Gladstone, who served four times as prime minister of England in the late nineteenth century, did a linguistic analysis of the works of Homer and found that the colors most frequently men-tioned were black and white. Other colors were clearly wrong: sheep described as violet, for example, or fearful human faces as green. Most strikingly, however, Homer never used the word *blue*. In his writings, as is well known, the sea is enigmatically described as "wine dark." Subsequent study revealed that blue is similarly missing from other ancient texts, including the Bible. The sky is most frequently described as white. Only later did words for blue appear. It seems that in order for the color to be seen, the word for it had to exist first. This surprising conclu-sion has subsequently been verified by modern scientific ex-perimentation.[1]

Apparently, in at least some cases, the brain has to be able to understand something before it can see or hear it. Sensory information is not transmitted and passively received, register-ing somewhere in our minds. Rather, our minds actively seek it, and put their stamp on it in the very process of registering that it is there. In chapter 2 I described how different things sounded to me after I had a large buildup of wax removed from my ears, and the gradual adjustment by which my hearing re-turned to "normal." The only thing really remarkable about this experience was that it made me aware of the way my brain was retuning my hearing. Most of the time it is making large adjust-ments to the information it receives from my ears and I don't notice anything remarkable happening—and that is exactly the point.

Here is how audiologist Marshall Chasin describes the way we come to understand pitch:

> When a sound is heard, the brain records which [hair cells in the cochlea] are stimulated and makes an initial guess as to the pitch of the sound. Then the brain "turns off" OHC's [outer hair cells] in areas just adjacent to the "best guess" critical band. If the amount of nerve impulse stays the same, then the brain knows that the majority of the sound must have come from the best guess critical band. If, however, the amount of nerve impulse is reduced, then those adjacent areas must also contain significant energy and sound.
>
> After a few of these "call and response" runs, the brain has a very accurate idea of the frequency of the sound, and then forms a perception of pitch.[2]

All of this happens within a fraction of a second and below the level of consciousness; all we are aware of hearing is what our brain finally decides is the correct pitch. A further complication arises from the fact that most notes are actually complex tones consisting of a fundamental and overtones, also known as harmonics or partials. "To extract the pitch, the auditory system must somehow combine and synthesize information from these harmonics. Exactly how this occurs in the auditory system remains a matter of ongoing research."[3]

Of course pitch is only one of the most basic elements of sound. To fully understand the sounds we hear, we must also bring conscious thought into the picture, and we often make use of the other senses as well. Suppose you drive down a busy city street while taking in the complex mixture of noises you would expect to encounter there. In all likelihood this includes the engine of your own car, your car's interaction with the surface of the street, and the sounds of other cars passing, perhaps with music emanating from inside. It may include louder engine noises coming from a passing bus or an airplane flying overhead. Sirens from emergency vehicles may approach or recede in the distance. At any point, each of these sounds is either growing louder or softer as the vehicle that produces it draws closer or moves farther away. And there may be other noises as well, some of which come from stationary sources. This is a complex sonic environment, and your brain will work hard to make sense of it, drawing on information from your eyes in the process. The sound of the bus, for example, will separate and come into prominence if the bus approaches from a side street and crosses in front of you while you are stopped at a light. Your knowledge of where you are—at a crowded intersection with many moving vehicles—will help you make this distinction and allow you not to be alarmed by sounds that in a different environment might produce fear and cause you to flee.

What you hear, in other words, is inseparable from where you are and what your mind and your other senses tell you about your surroundings. Your ability to interpret the sounds of a city street depends on your knowledge of cities and your previous experience with them. Someone from an isolated society who had never been in a city before would find these sounds much more difficult to interpret, even with the help of his or her eyes.

Music works much the same way. Someone who has never heard music in a particular style is unlikely to know what to make of it at first. Even music students take ear-training courses in order to fine-tune their perceptions of the music they know best. Unlike a city street, though, music contains sounds that are generated for their own sake and do not coordinate directly to meaning. When you hear a bus go by, your understanding of the sound is complete when you figure out what is producing it and how the bus's presence affects you. Knowing how a musical sound is produced is not as important as making musical sense of what you are hearing—a fact attested to by the large number of people who experience music primarily through audio recordings. It is entirely possible to enjoy a recording of an instrument one has never seen or heard before without knowing what the instrument looks like or how it is constructed. For example, you may hear a Japanese *koto* and think, "That sounds like a harp," without having any idea that the *koto*, unlike the harp, has strings that are arranged horizontally. While this is interesting to know and would be evident during a live performance, it does not affect your experience of the recorded music—nor does it need to. But your understanding of *koto* music would be augmented considerably by study of the instrument's repertoire and the different playing styles it calls for.

If listening to music is a skill acquired through practice and experience, performing and writing music are even more so. Most musicians begin studying their craft as children, and the greatest ones often start at a very young age. Recent research has suggested that musical training during childhood has substantial benefits that not only persist throughout life but also extend beyond music. Those who were trained in music as children are more likely to have perfect pitch. They are also better able to distinguish speech from background noise as they grow older. They are often better readers. These benefits can be traced to the way musicians' brains understand auditory information.[4]

Research on the way the brain processes sound has flourished in the quarter century since the publication of Albert Bregman's book *Auditory Scene Analysis* in 1990. Bregman, a Canadian psychologist, had been studying hearing perception for much of his career, taking advantage of modern technology that allowed him to control his subjects' auditory experiences with great precision. Bregman hypothesized that we use the signals we receive from our ears to form an "auditory scene," just as we create a visual scene with our eyes. As he explained, forming such a scene is fraught with difficulties:

> Imagine that you are on the edge of a lake and a friend challenges you to play a game. The game is this: Your friend digs two narrow channels up from the side of the lake. Each is a few feet long and a few inches wide and they are spaced a few feet apart. Halfway up each one, your friend stretches a handkerchief and fastens it to the sides of the channel. As waves reach the side of the lake they travel up the channels and cause the two handkerchiefs to go into motion. You are allowed to look only at the handkerchiefs and from their motions to answer a series of questions: How many boats are there on the lake and where are they? Which is the most powerful one? Which one is closer? Is the wind blowing? Has any large object been dropped suddenly into the lake?[5]

The channels are our ear canals, and the handkerchiefs are our eardrums. The lake is the air, and its waves are sound waves. The challenge Bregman describes captures the elusiveness of auditory information: the sheer amount of interpretation that needs to be done in order to make sense of what we hear.[6]

By contrast, the visual scene that surrounds us may seem self-explanatory. If you are looking at the lake Bregman describes, the boats will be easy to count, their positions immediately discernible. There will be no need for channels and handkerchiefs. According to this analogy, hearing gives us only indirect information about things that our eyes see directly.

The reality is much more complicated, of course. What we see is also limited by what our eyes can record and our brains can understand. Is the lake's water blue? Perhaps not to the ancient Greeks. Is the wind blowing? Unless the boats are sail-boats, it can be hard to tell by looking at them. The informa-tion we get from our eyes still leaves much for us to interpret. Hearing, meanwhile, is not really like watching handkerchiefs and observing their motions. Just as with vision, much of the work our ears perform happens automatically. We then learn to impose schemas on the information we receive, allowing us to interpret it further based on experience. Such schema-based analysis is what enables us to make sense of a complex, noisy environment like a city street. It is what makes it possible for us to understand conversation in the midst of multiple distrac-tions. It is also what makes it possible for us to hear and enjoy music.[7]

On the other hand, if Bregman is correct, our brains are hard-wired to group similar sounds together and hear them as coming from a single source without the need to construct schemas to understand what we are hearing. All composers must work both with and against this and other primitive or-ganizing features of human hearing, which can be assumed to be the same in all cultures and historical periods.[8] An example of such a feature, which can be easily demonstrated under con-trolled laboratory conditions, is what he calls the "streaming ef-fect." When subjects hear an alternation of high and low tones played in quick succession, they tend to hear not a single series of pitches but two different ones occurring simultaneously. The faster the pitches are played or the farther apart they are in pitch, the more likely this is to occur.[9] Even if listeners are try-ing to hear all the pitches as a single sequence, there is a point at which it becomes impossible to do so. This is because the brain's primitive mechanisms produce the perception of two separate streams automatically. When pitches remain close to-gether, however, a listener may still be able to separate a single stream from the surrounding pitches through conscious effort.

This ability is an example of schema-based understanding that is learned rather than innate.[10]

Often a composer will take advantage of the primitive streaming effect to produce compellingly effective music in which consecutive notes appear to separate into two different streams of sound. It is particularly easy to do this with string instruments, since string players can easily alternate between strings to produce what can sound like two different melodies, each moving at half the prevailing tempo. On other instruments this would be more awkward, although the effect can easily be imitated at the piano. In the Preludio of his Violin Partita in E Major (example 6.1), J. S. Bach has the violinist play a nearly steady stream of sixteenth notes, but the effect is often that of two melodies being played at the same time. (As the above description suggests, this becomes more noticeable the faster the music is played.) However, Bach also includes passages of successive notes that can be heard only as fast-moving scales or arpeggios. The constant perceptual shift thus produced between a single auditory stream and two separate ones is the most notable feature of this movement. Like many composers, Bach shows an inherent understanding of how human hearing works and takes creative advantage of that knowledge.

It is important to note that these effects can be seen as well as heard. Bregman confirms that the way the ear links auditory streams is similar to the way the eye links images. Groups of items that are close to each other but far from other groups tend to be seen as belonging together, just as pitches that are close to each other but far from other pitches tend to be heard as separate streams.[11] The passages in example 6.1 where separate streams are heard, such as that beginning at measure 9, also look like they contain two separate lines of notes, while those that sound like a single line, such as measures 4 and 6–8, look that way as well. In this case, our eyes and our ears tell us the same thing.

But can the eyes develop novel ways of constructing a musi-

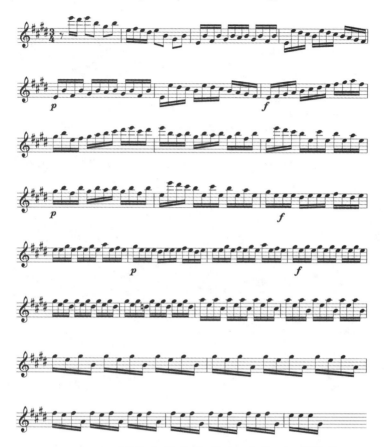

EXAMPLE 6.1. J. S. Bach, Violin Partita no. 3 in E major, Preludio,
mm. 1–26 (modified to show the notes as they sound)

cal scene that the ears will respond to as well? We have already
looked at numerous instances in which Beethoven seems to
have let his eyes take the lead while composing. Let us now
examine a short passage from the second movement of the Piano Sonata in F Major, op. 10, no. 2 (Example 6.2). Beethoven
probably wrote this piece in 1796, at precisely the point when
he began to be aware that he was losing his hearing. Composer
Jay Alan Zimmerman has even suggested that the first signs of
Beethoven's high-frequency hearing loss can be detected in the

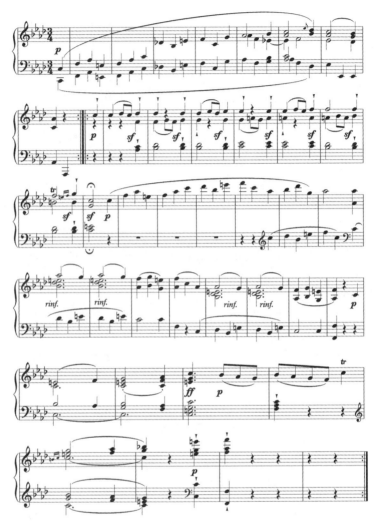

EXAMPLE 6.2. Beethoven, Piano Sonata in F Major,
op. 10, no. 2, 2nd movement, mm. 1–38

three sonatas of Opus 10, which repeatedly emphasize the bass register in a way not found in his earlier music.[12] But deliberate and original manipulation of keyboard textures can be found in both Beethoven's earliest and his latest works. Playing complicated games with the sound of the piano was a lifelong preoccupation of his.

This movement begins with both hands playing a broadly spaced melody in octaves that rises from the depths of the keyboard into its most melodic register. At the exact midpoint of the melody, everything about it changes: it begins to include half notes and an appoggiatura as well as quarter notes; the harmony shifts from bare octaves to full chords; and the long phrase mark that covers the first six measures gives way to two crisply articulated measures at the end. These stark shifts are accentuated by the contrast between the very low starting pitches and the much higher ones later on: a contrast that would have been even more pronounced on the pianos of Beethoven's time, with their rich, sonorous bass register and clear, bell-like treble. Beethoven seems to be challenging the listener to hear this heterogeneous material as a single auditory event, but he also presents a challenge to the performer, who must find a way to underscore the contrasts that are written into the music without exaggerating them to the point of incoherence.

After the repeat, the upper fingers of the right hand play a simple rhythmic figure three times in a row on successively higher pitches, separated by rests. Meanwhile, the right hand's lower fingers play the same succession of pitches a fifth lower and a measure behind, so that it fills up the gaps left by the upper notes. The left-hand accompaniment adds an offbeat accent to the beginning of each repetition. Following the fermata, the right hand plays the movement's opening melody in the highest register of Beethoven's piano. A spooky pianissimo imitation of the melody finally enters in the left hand, only to migrate into successively lower octaves as the bass line of a fully harmonized cadential phrase (mm. 23–30). The two hands then conclude the section in a standard melody and accompaniment texture, which stands out precisely because it has not been heard up to this point.

These frequent changes of texture continually challenge us to reassess the nature of the auditory event we are experiencing. Each time we think we have grasped where the melody is and how it relates to the accompaniment, Beethoven throws us a new surprise—and the surprises continue in the second part of the movement, in which a steady supporting octave in the bass suddenly morphs into a prominent melodic line in its own right (mm. 55–70).

In crafting the passage shown in example 6.2, Beethoven showed an intuitive knowledge of facts about hearing that have since received scientific support. The melody begins with widely spaced notes and large intervals (including the tritone), which research by Bregman and others has shown are harder for the ear to link into a single auditory stream than conjunct, or successive, notes like those with which the melody concludes.[13] The second four measures thus serve as a foil to the first four. The independence of the short melodic fragments in the right hand in measures 9–14 is heightened by the placement of rests, causing each "voice" to go silent at precisely the point where the other one is most active. The strong dissonant downbeats in measures 23, 24, 27, and 28 give extra weight and coherence to the penultimate phrase, causing us to hear the right hand as the melody even though the left hand is playing melodic material we have heard several times previously.

How did Beethoven know to do these things? Some of them are simple common sense: an accented right-hand melody will always stand out; rhythmically staggered canonic imitations had been written many times before. The strongly contrasting registers of the Viennese pianos on which he played would have made some of the contrasts he introduced even more striking; Beethoven went up to the highest note available on most such pianos and nearly down to the lowest. As with the Bach partita, though—and perhaps even more so—the effects Beethoven employed in this music are evident to the eye as well as to the ear. The contrasts of register and articulation in example 6.2 are visually striking. Long slurs encase the first six measures on both sides; the one for the right hand begins in the lower staff and rises over the upper one. The hands begin playing together in the lower staff, leaving the upper one empty, so the music may appear lopsided. Beethoven's experiments with the writing process, which puzzled Joseph Kerman in his study of the early sketches (see chapter 3), seem to have borne strange and exotic fruit. Kerman's edition of the *Kafka Miscellany*, which contains the only known sketches for opus 10, suggests that this movement germinated from a brief eight-measure fragment on a single staff (fig. 9) that contains some of its most interesting features: the long slurs, the dramatic contrast of registers, and the alternation of two distinct voices, each of which sounds when the other rests. All of these things are clearly visible here, even though this fragment contains none of the movement's distinctive melodic material. Intriguingly, that material first appeared on the other side of the same sketch page (fig. 10), but minus the slurs, the dramatic rise from the bass register, and the rhythmically alternating voices. We can speculate that Beethoven grafted these in as the movement developed into its final form, perhaps going back to the piano and incorporating features that had first occurred to him in writing. Even at this stage in his life, he knew how to let his eyes take the lead.

If Beethoven was composing with his eyes at age twenty-five, it is only logical to assume that he drew on this ability more and

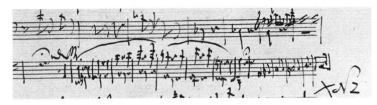

FIGURE 9. Preliminary sketch for the second movement
of op. 10, no. 2, in the Kafka miscellany

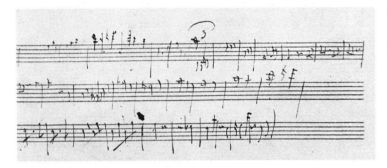

FIGURE 10. The top of the other side of the same page in the
Kafka Miscellany, showing the melodic material that Beethoven
fit into the framework sketched earlier. Source: Joseph Kerman,
ed., *Ludwig van Beethoven, Autograph Miscellany from Circa 1786
to 1799: British Museum Additional Manuscript No. 29801, ff. 39–
162 (The Kafka Sketchbook)* (London: British Museum, 1970).

more as his hearing grew worse. Just as someone with hearing
loss may rely increasingly on lipreading to understand speech,
whether consciously or unconsciously, so Beethoven would
have increasingly realized that his pen was a powerful supple-
ment to his failing ears.

There is no single story of hearing loss; it is something that is
experienced differently by each person. Like Beethoven, Barbara lost her hearing gradually beginning in her mid-twenties,
but for her the onset of total deafness was sudden. Unlike Bee-

thoven, she spent a few years deaf in one ear and not the other, which meant she had no depth perception of the auditory scene around her. Without it, she was unable to tell from what direction sounds were approaching, which could make something as simple as taking a walk in our sidewalk-free neighborhood a frightening experience; a car in the distance would not reveal its location until it was practically upon her.

Barbara did not compose music and did not play an instrument, but music had always been important to her; it was all the more so after she married me, since much of our social life together centered on going to concerts and singing in choirs. Thus regaining the ability to hear music was a very high priority for her. The technology at her disposal was very different from that available to Beethoven, but like Beethoven, she discovered that it opened up doors that had previously been shut, and that was reason enough to persist.

Barbara often said, "The human brain is an amazing thing." She wasn't speaking of reasoning ability or what most people would call "intelligence." What she meant was that, based on her own experience, the physical wiring of the brain could adapt to changes in sensory input. This didn't mean that those changes were immediate or comprehensive. It did mean that they could be transformative for those who experienced them.

Earlier I described the trip that Barbara and I made in the mid-1990s to be fitted for a hearing aid by John Berry, owner of the Blount Hearing and Speech Center in Maryville, Tennessee. What we learned from him transformed our understanding of hearing loss and the plasticity of the adult brain. Following the pathbreaking, but currently unfashionable, work of Peter Guberina, John believes that both children and adults can learn to hear better with only a small amount of auditory information, even if the ear itself does not change. This explains the improvement in Barbara's unaided speech recognition after we began using the pocket talker. Once she had learned to maximize her use of the information this "hearing machine" was providing, she could understand much more without it as well.[14]

That was not the case with the cochlear implants. In December 2005 Barbara became "bilateral," receiving a second implant in her right ear, which was activated the following month. The process of implantation destroyed the tiny amount of residual hearing that Barbara had left in that ear, which was what had enabled her to make such progress with the pocket talker. Once she disconnected her external processors for the night—she quickly learned to call them "my ears"—she was functionally deaf, and no amount of auditory information would have registered. With the implants, though, her brain made remarkable progress. Just a few weeks after hookup of her second implant she wrote:

> I just had a very unexpected but exciting thing happen to me. I had just arrived home from taking my kids to gym when the phone rang. During my drive, the battery on my left CI (my older one) went out. So I only had my right one working at the time. . . . I answered the phone not knowing if I could hear anything or not. It was my mom and I could identify that it was her! And that was on my new side! I quickly went to my bedroom to change batteries so I could carry on a conversation with her. But it was so exciting to me to actually hear her talk on the phone with my new CI![15]

Simply talking on the phone with an implant is a leap for many people. Identifying a voice without being able to see who is speaking is also a challenge. It had taken Barbara months to be able to do either of these things after implantation on the left. Thus she was startled and gratified to find that in less than a month her perception of voices with the new implant had advanced sufficiently that she was able to identify her mother on the phone with her right ear. She still needed her left ear to carry on a conversation, though, because she had had much more practice listening to words with the older implant, and that ear was useless until she put in a new battery. As soon as the current began to flow, she received the benefit of that progress, which clearly did not transfer to the right ear; just as it had on the left, her speech comprehension in that ear would have to progress more gradually.

We initially anticipated that Barbara's perception of music would progress in a similar fashion, gradually reaching the point where music could sound almost normal. At the cochlear implant users' group in Dallas we had spoken to people who were able to play instruments and enjoy live music. There seemed to be no reason not to hope that Barbara would be able to return to singing in a choir a few years down the road. We soon came to understand, though, that the CI is designed to facilitate the understanding of speech, not music. As one researcher has put it:

> CIs do not transmit a faithful representation of musical sounds. Rather, CIs transmit those acoustic features considered most salient to speech perception. . . . The speech processor stimulation rates are unrelated to the precise frequency components of the input signals. Providing only gross spectral information to implant users is adequate for perception of segmental features of speech in quiet, as well as rhythmic (durational) components of music.
>
> The coarse spectral information of the signal is problematic, however, with regard to perception of pitch and timbre, two of the most important structural attributes of music.[16]

The perception of pitch depends on being able to identify frequencies that are very close together as separate notes; there are eighty-eight such notes on a standard piano keyboard, and even higher and lower ones are audible as separate pitches. Implants stimulate the cochlea using a much smaller range of discrete channels—Barbara's had sixteen—and they deliver those signals only to the outer end of the cochlea, which is accustomed to hearing the highest pitches. There is no reason such impoverished auditory information should enable someone to hear discrete pitches at all, let alone yield a truly satisfying musical experience. Adjacent notes like C, D, and E might all come in on the same electrode and stimulate the exact same spot on the cochlea. Logic would seem to dictate that an implant user would never be able to distinguish between notes so close together.[17] Strangely, though, Barbara often could, and many other implant users have been able to do so as well.

Timbre, the quality of a sound, is even more complicated. One of its major determinants is the overtone structure of the fundamental pitch: which higher notes vibrate together with it at multiples of the original frequency. In order to hear timbre correctly, the ear must distinguish not just one pitch but several. Most people do this automatically; they are not aware of the overtones as separate pitches but simply hear one note with a particular tone quality. An implant user, though, cannot easily make the kinds of distinctions that the perception of timbre requires. For this reason it may be hard to hear a series of pitches as a melody or to tell which instrument is playing them.

Furthermore, research has suggested that the kind of primitive auditory scene analysis needed to make sense of music, including the streaming effect, which is hard-wired into the brains of people with normal hearing, cannot be assumed to function in people with cochlear implants. For this reason they need to rely on learned experience to make even the most basic musical distinctions, so that music listening becomes for them a much more mentally demanding task.[18]

Given these limitations, it seems remarkable that cochlear implant users are able to enjoy music at all. What the experiences of Barbara and many others demonstrate is that memory and visual associations can help stimulate the brain to "hear" far more than the signals from the implant might seem to suggest. Just as I could perceive a car alarm from my basement office only once I knew what it was I was listening to, so implant users apparently fill in the blanks from stored musical memories, sometimes aided by visual cues. Arlene Romoff, who has documented her CI experience in two books, writes of attending the movie *Titanic* after receiving her first implant. Although much of the music was confusing, "the string quartet, playing on the deck of the *Titanic*, sounded like a string quartet. Perhaps also because it looked like a string quartet. Just a guess here, that by *seeing* strings, my brain is more inclined to *hear* strings."[19]

People with profound hearing loss, like Beethoven, can have similar experiences without cochlear implants. "I equate it to muscle memory," writes singer Ali Zimmerman, who lost her hearing in her mid-twenties. "If you break your leg and can't walk for weeks, when you are healed your muscles will remember what to do and with enough exercise you'll be able to walk again. I learned that if I exercised my hearing with music that I knew prior to my hearing loss, I would be able to hear it. It was simply a matter of training my brain to reinterpret the signals it was getting."[20]

Barbara had many comparable experiences. Usually understanding would break through suddenly, in what she came to call "CI moments." Just a few days after her initial hookup she was able to recognize a few familiar Christmas carols at a Christmas Eve church service. This would not have been possible if she had not known in advance that they were going to be sung. Less than six months later, she was surprised and delighted when she was able to recognize a familiar hymn on her own.

> I had a wonderful, surprising CI moment in church today. During communion, they were singing some hymns. They were noted in the bulletin only by page numbers; not by name. I wasn't following in my hymnal so had no way of knowing beforehand what they were playing. All of a sudden, I recognized the tune they were playing and knew what it was! . . . Our organ is way at the back of the church in a loft and I have never been able to follow any tune she was playing before. I left church with a huge grin on my face![21]

At the end of that year we attended a singalong performance of Handel's *Messiah*, a piece Barbara had performed several times and knew extremely well. She happily reported, "I was able to sing most everything and even come in when I was supposed to! I don't know how good I sounded, but that doesn't really matter. Just the fact that I could sing the notes, count my cues, and come in when I was supposed to was a miracle in itself."[22] Unfortunately, Barbara was not able to repeat this experience with other music, and her dream of once again singing in a choir slowly faded.

Barbara's mental Rolodex of stored musical memories yielded hits primarily when she was able to recognize a melody; her brain would then apparently fill in the rest, even though the signal from the implant could not provide the degree of pitch discrimination that hearing a new and unfamiliar melody would require. She wasn't incapable of learning new melodies, but doing so required enormous concentration.

Other cochlear implant users with extensive musical training have also had breakthrough moments when old, established hearing schemas apparently asserted themselves unconsciously, making things sound completely different than they had just a few moments before. Lindy Crocker, a sixty-year-old Australian pianist, began to lose her hearing in her thirties and received an implant a few years ago. At first, she says, she relied heavily on her memory of what it felt like to produce a good tone. "I would check my hand and finger positions often, knowing that they were true and anticipate the sound I was producing. I started playing easy pieces that I knew very very well. Also, due to my musicianship, I knew in my mind what the sound should be like (pitch wise) even though the CI processor hadn't caught up yet."[23] Later, she says, when playing more complicated pieces in public, she was taken aback when the first notes she played sounded atonal; she was not only hearing the wrong notes but hearing them in a way that negated any sense of higher-level pitch organization. (Barbara had the same experience shortly after hookup when she reported that a performance of piano music by Beethoven and Brahms sounded "modern.") In less than a minute, though, the sound would suddenly shift and she would hear it correctly. Like many aspects of hearing with implants, this improved over time, but

occasionally, I hear atonal sounds or sounds at the wrong pitch and then in a few seconds/moments the sound becomes true. It was a little off putting of course but I mostly smiled inwardly, glad that no-one else could hear this and felt grateful and relieved when the proper sounds came. Not sure why this happens but I believe my brain is "kicking in" to the sounds it knew once, or my music intelligence takes over perhaps. . . .

When listening to known music I hear mostly what I expect to hear, or do after a few phrases or bars. When it is new music, I struggle more to "understand" what is happening. If I have the score in front of me then I do much

much better—knowing how it should sound from the score and then the brain 'kicks in.'[24]

The sense of the brain "kicking in," suddenly providing a new level of understanding that was unavailable seconds earlier, is apparently widely shared by implant users, and perhaps by other people with severe hearing loss as well. Many also testify to the importance of physical experiences: touch at the keyboard, the way the head, mouth, and nasal cavity feel while singing,[25] the position of the fingers while playing a string instrument. All of these can serve not just as connections with the past but as bridges that help the brain to hear better in the present. As the experiences of Barbara and others suggest, they can also help to rewire the brain, just as the pocket talker did, and lead to better hearing even without any physiological change to the ear.

Even in the absence of such dramatic changes, careful preparation and vigilant watching can help people with hearing loss feel more confident, allowing them to perform in ensembles and sometimes even lead them. Many people have read Louis Spohr's dismissive description of Beethoven's conducting at the time of the premiere of the Seventh Symphony in 1813. According to Spohr, during one of the rehearsals Beethoven ignored a fermata and got several measures ahead of the orchestra, then appeared startled when he realized they were not playing *forte* as he expected.[26] There is a less-known account of the same performances written by an anonymous member of the orchestra that is much more revealing.

Beethoven may still have been able to hear the tuttis, and he held them together through the heavenly fire of his expression and gestures in beating time. He directed the more delicate sections calmly and with a soulful expression, as though he heard everything, and the meticulous rehearsals that the orchestra had carried out with inexhaustible perseverance lifted the performance to a ravishing perfection. During the performance, I noticed that when Beethoven did not feel entirely sure of himself in following certain figurations in the violins, he watched Schuppanzigh's bowing and beat time accordingly.[27]

A similar experience is recounted by Joan Ernst, a former music teacher with severe hearing loss who has nevertheless been able to serve as a church choir director.

When I am directing, I am reading the music and know what it should sound like. I try to convey that in my directing and it seems to work. The choir members know of my limitations and work with me. Through lip reading and body language, I can perceive what is happening and notice mistakes—especially rhythmic ones. But I cannot tell if someone sings the wrong note at the right time. They are on the honor system to tell me if they are not getting the right notes. My husband, who has an excellent ear for music, sings tenor from the back row and often gives me visual cues when someone is off.[28]

Like Beethoven, Ernst relies on the dedication of her ensemble and uses visual cues from them to make sure she is holding things together. When necessary, her eyes become a substitute for her ears. The result is a challenging, frustrating, but occasionally also rewarding experience, as we can imagine conducting the premiere of the Seventh Symphony was for Beethoven.

We have already seen that Beethoven became accustomed as a young man to using the physical act of writing and the visual appearance of his scores to generate musical ideas, not just to record them. Timothy Polashek, a composer and music technology professor with a lifelong hearing loss, suggests that "musicians with hearing loss are drawn to music because you have to think about it a little more." Polashek relates that as a child he was often unable to understand speech, so he was forced to pay more attention to the rhythm and tone of the human voice, which naturally led to an interest in music.[29] When Beethoven found that he could no longer take his hearing for granted, he was prepared to use his sketches and manuscripts as anchors, allowing him to return to a safe harbor even while exploring uncharted waters in his newest works. Perhaps one reason he valued his early sketches so highly, taking them with him during the dozens of moves he made later in life, is that they provided a kind of physical Rolodex that helped his brain to kick in, generating new ideas that were then added to his ever-expanding base of source material. Every so often he would reach into the earliest layers and repurpose something that had lain dormant for decades, as when he drew the first theme of his final piano sonata, Opus 111, completed in 1822, from a draft first made twenty years earlier in 1801–2.[30] At other times he used the touch and feel of the keyboard as his anchor, which helps explain why he also brought a piano to every new residence, including his summer decampments to the countryside, even after his hearing loss became profound.

Beethoven's success can be measured by the fact that he not only continued composing but ventured further and further afield as his deafness grew. Is it possible that the extraordinary creativity of his middle and late periods took place not despite his deafness but because of it? By looking closely at the way he created the music on which his reputation rests, we can see how he used both writing and the keyboard to nudge new sounds and textures into existence, perhaps inadvertently rewiring not just his own musical brain but those of generations to come. As his failing ears increasingly forced his eyes into the driver's seat, he created new musical textures and new approaches to musical form, forever changing the experience of music for those who came after him.

* 7 *

Hearing through the Eyes

In his pioneering book *Extraordinary Measures: Disability in Music,* Joseph Straus writes with great insight about the fourteenth-century Italian composer Francesco Landini (ca. 1325–97), whose extraordinary musical creativity, much like Homer's ability to tell an epic story with great poetic skill, was attributed by his contemporaries to the blindness that had afflicted him since childhood. "Yet I think it might be productive to think again about Landini's blindness in relation to his music," Straus writes,

> and it might be best to begin by thinking about how his music was actually, physically composed. In Landini's time, the late medieval period, musical composition generally involved memory and improvisation. Composers did not jot down musical sketches, then notate successive versions of a musical work, leading to a final score from which individual vocal or instrumental parts could be extracted. . . . Rather, composition routinely took place in the memory, in interaction with vocal or instrumental improvisation. At some point, the work would be notated, either by the composer or by a scribe working at the composer's behest. Landini was famous both for his prodigious

memory and for his skill as an improviser and, according to contemporary observers, his abilities in both areas were enhanced by his blindness. Indeed, one might say that his blindness enabled him to do more successfully the crucial things that all composers of his day were expected to do.[1]

By Beethoven's time this had changed completely. Although improvisation was still important—a point I have emphasized throughout this book—composers like Haydn and Mozart increasingly relied on sketching and revising their works, arriving at the finished version much as a painter sketches the form of a finished work and then gradually fills it in.

Beethoven has long since become a classic. His innovations are now mainstream, and we can no more hear them the way they sounded to their first listeners than we can have the experience of hearing a steam engine or a grand piano for the first time. Fortunately we can still watch Beethoven at work. In his manuscripts and sketches we can see his ideas taking shape, and with a little imagination our eyes can help uncover their novelty. In many cases Beethoven appears to have been formulating not just musical themes and structures but sounds and textures as well. He was also indulging a lifelong preoccupation of his: that "veritable commitment to the graphic act" that Joseph Kerman noted even in his earliest sketches. It seems to have been very important to him to see what he was doing: to work out ideas visually and not just make notes of what he had heard or played. Indeed, writing as a creative act is what Beethoven's sketches and manuscripts record, and by looking at them carefully we can get a sense of it as a physical process through which he pulled music out of the world of sound and firmly into the parallel worlds of sight and touch.

The two excerpts from the collection of early Beethoven sketches known as the *Kafka Miscellany* shown in figures 11 and 12 never made it into a finished work, but they give an idea of

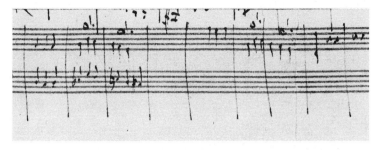

FIGURE 11. A sketch for an unfinished piano fantasy on folio 93 verso of the Kafka Miscellany. Source: Joseph Kerman, ed., *Ludwig van Beethoven, Autograph Miscellany from circa 1786 to 1799: British Museum Additional Manuscript no. 29801, ff. 39–162 (The Kafka Sketchbook)* (London: British Museum, 1970).

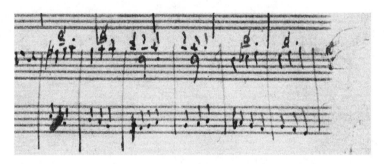

FIGURE 12. Another passage from the same series of sketches on folio 94 verso of the Kafka Miscellany. Source: Joseph Kerman, ed., *Ludwig van Beethoven, Autograph Miscellany from circa 1786 to 1799: British Museum Additional Manuscript no. 29801, ff. 39–162 (The Kafka Sketchbook)* (London: British Museum, 1970).

why it is important to look carefully at what Beethoven was doing. They are from a part of the collection with a distinct paper type that probably dates from 1795, when Beethoven was at work on the Second Piano Concerto, op. 19, and before he began noticing symptoms of hearing loss.[2] Both are fragments that probably belong to the last movement of an unfinished three-movement piano work in D minor; they are shown in transcription in example 7.1.[3] In almost every way they are unremarkable. Both are in 3/4 time and feature running quarter

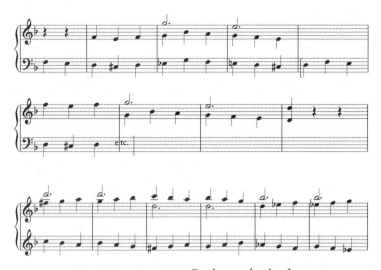

EXAMPLE 7.1A AND B. Beethoven, sketches for an
unfinished piano fantasy from the Kafka Miscellany

notes in both the right and left hands; in the first the quarter
notes move together in the same direction—what musicians
call parallel motion—and in the second they move in opposite
directions—known as contrary motion.

In both fragments, though, there is a third "voice" in the
right hand consisting of dotted half notes, each of which takes
up an entire measure. In modern notation, as shown by Joseph
Kerman's transcriptions of these passages in his edition of the
Kafka Miscellany,[4] these notes would be aligned vertically with
the first quarter note in each measure, yielding a three-note
chord of one beat's duration. In Beethoven's time, though—as
countless early printed editions make clear—it was customary to place a long note that occupied an entire measure in the
exact middle of the measure, ignoring vertical alignment with
the other notes. Beethoven followed this convention with the
dotted half notes in these sketches, making them align with the
second quarter note in each measure.

Modern musicians looking at Beethoven's notation may initially find it confusing. To play the music as it is apparently written, with a dotted quarter note on the second beat of each measure, one would have to ignore the bar lines and tolerate some strong harmonic clashes. While this was clearly not what Beethoven intended, the notational conventions of his time did encourage him to see and write the longer notes as physically separate from the others and hence as constituting a distinct auditory stream. When the higher stream in the second fragment leaps down an octave and then leaps back up two measures later, the dotted half notes and the quarter notes are still visibly set apart in Beethoven's sketch, whereas in the modern transcription the voices appear to have changed places: ♩♩♩|♩♩♩| dotted half | dotted half on the top and dotted half |dotted half |♩♩♩|♩♩♩ on the bottom. A musician today is prone to both see and hear this passage differently than Beethoven did, understanding and playing all the high notes into the melody and all the low notes into the accompaniment.

The lesson of this example is that Beethoven's writing—his physical notes—may convey important information about the music that may not be easily discernible by ear or even visible in his published scores, especially in modern editions. Like the sketch for Opus 10 discussed in the last chapter, and like the "very strange" early sketches that Joseph Kerman noticed fifty years ago, these sketches for an unfinished work show "a compulsion to get things down on paper." But they show more than that. They show that for Beethoven, paper was a laboratory for conceptualizing musical textures, especially ones that might present unusual challenges. The one he came up with in this case is almost too simple to merit special notice—a third voice emerging from a polyphonic texture would hardly seem novel to anyone accustomed to the often free voice leading of other eighteenth-century composers—but after he began to lose his hearing Beethoven would continue to experiment with visually interesting textures that brought his listeners to, and sometimes beyond, the limit of what they could easily absorb.

Consider the *Grosse Fuge*, op. 133, written in 1825–26 when Beethoven's deafness was at its most complete. This is widely recognized as his most radical work. Originally written as the finale of the String Quartet in B-flat Major, op. 130, it caused consternation at its first performance, leading Beethoven to write a new finale and publish the fugue as a separate work. The comments by the Viennese correspondent of the *Allgemeine musikalische Zeitung* on that first performance are worth quoting in full.

> The most recent quartet by Beethoven in B-flat (the third among the last ones), consisting of the following movements: *a*. Allegro moderato; *b*. Presto; *c*. Scherzo Andantino; *d*. Alla danza tedesca; *e*. Cavatina; *f*. Fuga. The first, third, and fifth movements are serious, gloomy, mystical, but also at times bizarre, rough, and capricious; the second and fourth full of mischief, good cheer, and roguishness. Here the great composer, who, particularly in his most recent works, has seldom known how to find appropriate limits, has expressed himself unusually briefly and convincingly. The repetition of both movements was demanded with stormy applause. But the reviewer does not dare to interpret the sense of the fugal finale; for him it was incomprehensible, like Chinese. If the instruments in the regions of the South and North Poles have to struggle with gigantic difficulties; if each of them is differently figured and they cross over each other *per transitum irregularem* amid countless dissonances; if the players, not trusting themselves, probably also do not play completely accurately, then the Babylonian confusion is certainly complete.

There then exists a concert at which Moroccans might possibly enjoy themselves—those who, during their presence at the Italian opera here, found nothing pleasing but the instruments harmonizing in empty fifths, and the customary preluding by all the instruments at once. Perhaps so much would not have been written down if the master were also able to hear his own creations. But we do not wish thereby to pronounce a negative judgment prematurely; perhaps the time is yet to come when that which at first glance appeared to us dismal and confused will be recognized as clear and pleasing in form.[5]

This report contains an early version of a story that has been repeated countless times since: that a visitor or visitors from a foreign musical culture enjoyed the tuning and warming up of a Western orchestra more than the actual performance that followed. The persistence of this fable is an ironic acknowledgment that Western listeners are accustomed to musical schemas that not everyone is prepared to grasp. The anonymous author, though, showed an acute understanding of the challenges of listening to the *Grosse Fuge*, which he understood to contain its own complex schemas that were unfathomable to him. The parts for the four instruments often clashed, yet they crossed over each other frequently; as a result, the way they blended struck him as confusing rather than harmonious, much like the melee of sounds emanating from an orchestra settling in before a performance.

Beethoven, the *Allgemeine musikalische Zeitung* correspondent believed, had relied too much on what the music looked like on paper and was unable to judge the results with his ears. The reviewer understood, though, that future audiences might reverse his judgment, just as they had overcome the bafflement initially produced by some of Beethoven's earlier works.

In 1799, for example, another writer in the *Allgemeine musikalische Zeitung* had greeted the sonatas of Opus 10 with the observation that Beethoven's imagination "too often still causes
him to pile up ideas without restraint and to arrange them by
means of a bizarre manner so as to bring about an obscure ar-
tificiality or an artificial obscurity, which is disadvantageous
rather than advantageous to the effect of the entire piece."[6] He
no doubt had passages like example 6.2 in mind.

Such complex auditory scenes are found throughout Opus 10,
initially making it hard for those accustomed to eighteenth-
century keyboard textures to grasp. By the time of the *Grosse
Fuge* Beethoven's early style was no longer startling. It took
something more radical to confuse listeners' ears in the 1820s.
In this case, the fugal subject itself appears to be carved out of
two separate auditory streams: two adjacent notes are followed
by a large leap and two more adjacent notes. Beethoven used
versions of this same subject in two other quartets, Opus 132
and 131, the works written, respectively, before and after Opus
130. The *Grosse Fuge*, though, is its apotheosis. It opens with an
Overtura in which the theme is first proclaimed *forte* in unison, three times in a row. Each statement features the defining leap in an upward direction, followed by a leap back down
and another one back up, producing a sequence of eight notes
in which a high and a low stream appear to be combined. The
sequence is then repeated twice in faster note values, followed
by two other passages in which the same jagged melodic line
is prominently featured (example 7.2).

The extreme fragmentation of this opening is unusual, a
kind of musical scene perhaps not encountered again until the
twentieth century. The theme itself is not unique; as David
Levy has pointed out, the jagged leap around which it is built is
an example of the *saltus duriusculus*, the "somewhat harsh leap"
defined by baroque theorists and used by Bach and others to

underscore ideas of pain and sinfulness.[7] What is truly unprecedented about the extended fugue that follows (mm. 30–158) is that this dual-stream melodic line is combined with an energetic counter-subject that also features large, regular leaps between registers.[8] Between them, the two subjects suggest four separate auditory streams, and after all the instruments enter the picture becomes even more daunting. There are many points at which multiple, simultaneous register jumps in all the instruments create a string-quartet texture unlike any previously imagined. The parts are so enmeshed with each other that it is hard to hear them as individual lines, even though it is clear to the eye who is playing what (example 7.3).

In order for it to make sense to the ears as well, a piece of music needs to provide enough cues for an educated listener to have a musically satisfying experience. Although the *Allgemeine musikalische Zeitung* correspondent hedged his bets by admitting that future listeners might disagree, he clearly believed that a deaf composer might be unable to provide such cues. He did not find them himself, and several later generations of listeners agreed. It was not until the twentieth century that the *Grosse Fuge* was acknowledged as a successful work, let alone a masterpiece. Stravinsky described it as an "absolutely contemporary piece of music that will be contemporary forever."[9] One hundred forty years after it was written, it was still being acknowledged for its novelty, so it is hardly surprising that at its first performance an educated listener should have judged it incomprehensible.

If the *Grosse Fuge* baffled audiences, the three "Razumovsky" quartets, op. 59, written in 1806 when Beethoven's hearing was in decline, divided them. An *Allgemeine musikalische Zeitung* correspondent reported in 1807 that the "Razumovskys" were "deep in conception and marvelously worked out, but not universally comprehensible, with the possible exception of the

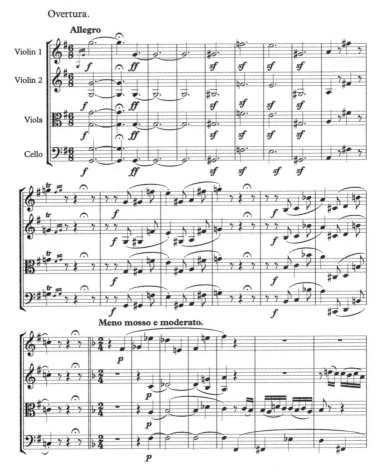

EXAMPLE 7.2. Beethoven, *Grosse Fuge* for String Quartet, op. 133, mm. 1–30 (up to the beginning of the section marked "Fuga")

third one, in C major, which by virtue of its individuality, melody, and harmonic power must win over every educated friend of music."[10]

In stating that the first two quartets were not universally comprehensible, this writer was drawing on his own observations of how the earliest audiences received them. Some in those

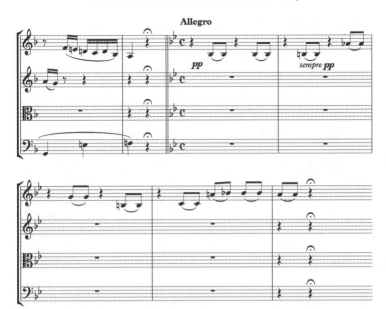

audiences, he suggested, were able to appreciate their deep conception and marvelous working out, while others were left baffled. What, specifically, would have confused them?

It could not simply have been the length of the "Razumovskys"; Beethoven had written even longer works that were more quickly assimilated than these. It could not have been the difficulty of performing these quartets; all three were extremely hard to play, but the third was judged more accessible. It could not have been extramusical meaning: none of them was complicated by a program or title, although the first two contained prominently marked Russian melodies in honor of Count Andreas Razumovsky, who commissioned them.

Nevertheless, there are features of the "Razumovsky" quartets—particularly the first, in F major—that make them markedly different from any previous music by Beethoven. These may be the works of his fourth decade in which

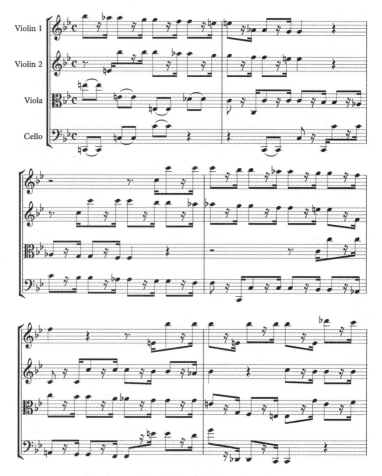

EXAMPLE 7.3. Beethoven, *Grosse Fuge* for String Quartet, op. 133, mm. 97–102

he showed the most notable musical response to his growing deafness, emphasizing features that could be felt physically by the musicians playing them and challenging his listeners' auditory imaginations with textures that appealed to the eyes as well as to the ears. His work on Opus 59, like that on Opus 18 eight years earlier, may have grown from an intuitive awareness that he needed to learn new ways of writing while he could still hear well enough to judge the results with his ears. Throughout the first quartet of Opus 59, and to a lesser degree in the second as well, Beethoven seems to have been preoccupied with disruption of the auditory scene through striking contrasts of register and instrumentation. Listening to these works for the first time, someone accustomed to a traditional string-quartet sound would have been repeatedly challenged to make connections between things that were normally kept apart, often having to rethink the relationships between the members of the ensemble from one moment to the next.[11]

There are other features that may reflect Beethoven's hearing loss as well. The F major quartet is obsessively rhythmic, and rhythms are much easier than pitches for failing ears to discern. Its second movement is based on a four-measure pattern stated on a single pitch, while the last movement is dominated by intersecting dotted rhythms and syncopations. In both movements high and low instruments frequently toss pairs of sixteenth notes back and forth, intensifying the beat in a way that is not only physically exciting but also highly visible to the audience (example 7.4).

The third movement, meanwhile, showcases Beethoven's growing attention to the streaming effect. His developing awareness of it is visually evident in the score, even if the ways he used it are less confusing to the ear than those in the *Grosse Fuge*. Fortunately, Beethoven's manuscript for this work has survived. As is so often the case, it contains extensive revisions and corrections, showing that Beethoven was still at work on the music as he wrote out the final version. Many of the changes he made had to do with the texture: the spacing of the parts and their relationship to one another, which more than anything else determines the nature of the auditory scene.

Example 7.5 begins at measure 23 and shows the second, contrasting theme of the movement's sonata structure as it

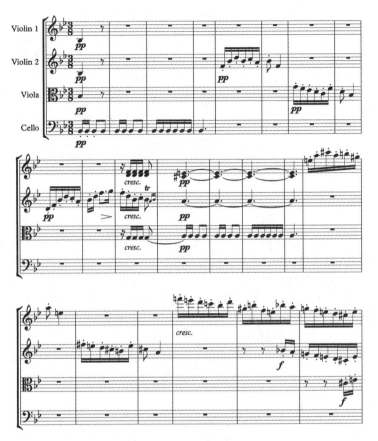

EXAMPLE 7.4. Beethoven, String Quartet in F Major, op. 59,
no. 1 ("Razumovsky no. 1"), 2nd movement, mm. 68–99

appears in the finished work. The first violin leads off with a
series of thirty-second notes that pivot around G_4, the G above
middle C; this pitch falls throughout on the even-numbered
notes of the series. Meanwhile, the accented, odd-numbered
notes trace two ascending G7 chords: first major, then minor.
Because of the streaming effect we hear this as a melody in sixteenth notes with a sustained G in the middle, rather than as a
succession of thirty-second notes.

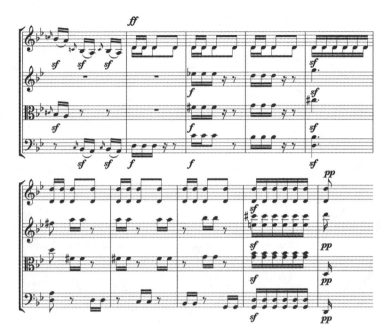

In measure 24 the cello begins playing the theme, which outlines a C minor chord in eighth notes, followed by its dominant, a G7 chord, in measure 25. Meanwhile the implied melody in the violin changes to a mostly stepwise sequence—E-flat, C, B, C, B, C, D, E-flat | F, E-flat, D, C, B, D, A-flat, B—all constantly alternating with G_4. We hear a slow melody in the cello and another one in the violin going twice as fast, with G_4 as the common tone around which both center.

Beethoven confirms that this is what he wanted us to hear by writing the implied violin melody in the cello at measure 26 as a steady stream of sixteenth notes, while the violin takes over the eighth-note melody that the cello played earlier. Meanwhile the second violin begins its own thirty-second-note pattern, with G_4 still the pivot note. The viola enters with a measure of middle C, followed by nearly a measure of G_3. The

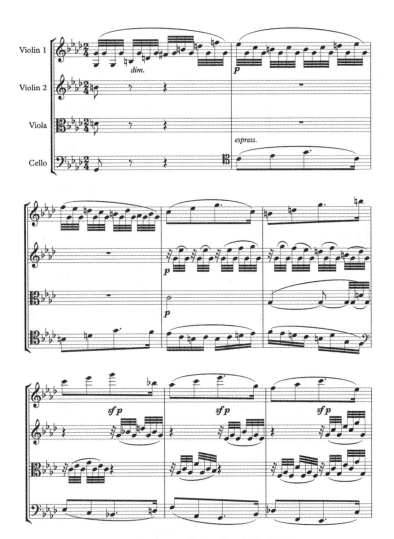

EXAMPLE 7.5. Beethoven, String Quartet in F Major, op. 59, no. 1 ("Razumovsky no. 1"), 3rd movement, mm. 23–30

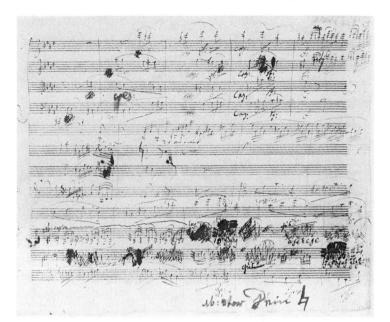

FIGURE 13. The bottom two systems of page 58 of Beethoven's
manuscript of the String Quartet in F Major, op. 59, no. 1. Source:
Alan Tyson, ed., Beethoven: *String Quartet Opus 59 No. 1 (First
"Razumovsky" Quartet, in F Major)* (London: Scolar, 1980).

resulting texture is one in which the four instruments play five
harmonic parts, two of them in the second violin.

Then, in measure 28, the first violin and cello both begin the
eighth-note melody, moving simultaneously in opposite directions while first the viola, then the second violin, accompany
them in thirty-second notes. This creates an implied six-part
texture for the next two measures, until the inner instruments
finally come together in parallel octaves in the second half of
measure 30.

The manuscript shows how much Beethoven struggled with
the layout of this passage (fig. 13). In measure 26 he seems to
have initially given the thirty-second notes to the viola with

G_3 as the pivot note, but he scratched them out and moved them to the second violin at the same pitch. Then he decided to move them up an octave using the octava sign—a decision he confirmed with a marginal note—bringing them into the same range as the first violin. He also apparently first intended the viola accompaniment to extend through measures 28 and 29 and to move parallel to the cello part. After some furious scratching out and rewriting, he was forced to indicate the final disposition of notes in the second violin and viola parts by writing out the letter names between the staves to make sure his intentions were clear.

All this revision once again shows Beethoven conceptualizing musical textures on paper. The end result is deceptively simple: a triadic melody that migrates from the bass to the treble; a pulsating countermelody pivoting around a note that lies between the two registers but corresponds to the cello's highest note; an expanding compass as bass and treble move into contrary motion, and the accompaniment reaches out in both directions. The process by which Beethoven arrived there, though, was by no means simple. His original impulse was to link the cello and viola parts from measure 26 through measure 30. As he moved the viola part up to the second violin stave, he seems to have realized that its upper stream was strong enough to stand in the same register as the violin, where it could function as a full-fledged countermelody and not simply a reinforcement of the cello part. The steady G which constituted the lower stream could then remain on G_4, where it would not be mistaken for the bass line in measure 26.

In 1806 Beethoven's hearing was still good enough for him to hear the results as well as see them on paper. More than two years later, it will be recalled, he made corrections in the score of the *Pastoral* Symphony after hearing the music performed. He must have been satisfied that the solution he came up with in this case not only looked good but sounded good as well.

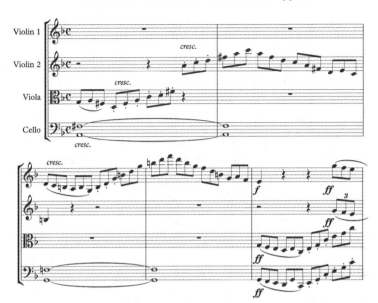

EXAMPLE 7.6. Beethoven, String Quartet in F Major, op. 59,
no. 1 ("Razumovsky no. 1"), 1st movement, mm. 79–83

Elsewhere in the first "Razumovsky" quartet he did more
radical things on paper, creating textures that must have struck
his first hearers as unnatural and contrary to the nature of the
string quartet. In measure 79 of the first movement a rising
triplet arpeggio leaps from the viola to the second violin on
beat 4 (example 7.6).

Because of the switch from alto to treble clef, the written
music here still looks like one continuous line. This is particularly clear in Beethoven's manuscript, because the note stems
on beat 3 in the viola are drawn upward, whereas every printed
edition, beginning with the first, has shown them going down-
ward. The print versions agree with notational convention
but break the visual continuity of the transition between the
two instruments, which Beethoven highlighted by the way he
wrote this passage.

A few measures later, beginning in measure 85, the ensemble

is fragmented in a different way: half notes in the violins on
high G and E are followed by half notes on C-sharp and A in the
viola and cello, two and a half octaves lower. Heard together—
and what choice does the listener have but to hear them that
way?—these produce a dominant seventh chord on A, which
does not resolve until five measures later in measure 90; it is
first succeeded by a G dominant seventh in the two violins in
the first half of m. 86 and an isolated low G in the cello in the
second half of that measure (example 7.7). The fragmentation
here is extreme. Not only is the ensemble broken up between
registers in a way that must have sounded nearly incoherent,
but two unresolved seventh chords are heard in succession and

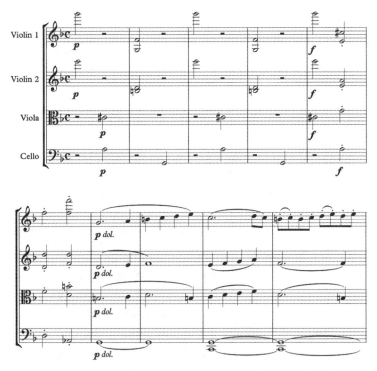

EXAMPLE 7.7. Beethoven, String Quartet in F major, op. 59,
no. 1 ("Razumovsky no. 1"), 1st movement, mm. 85–94

then repeated before the harmonic syntax is finally rationalized in measures 89–93.

This looks less radical on paper than it sounds. Because the violins are in treble clef and the viola and cello are in alto and bass clef, respectively, the spacing of the chords does not seem nearly as wide in the score as it is in actual fact. This doesn't mean, of course, that Beethoven didn't know what the effect he created would sound like. It does suggest, though, that both this and the viola-violin jump in measure 79 were by-products of the writing process. Both of these unusual passages originated as visual scenes. Beethoven didn't just let his eyes take the lead; in these cases he wrote music that may make more sense on paper than it does in performance. It is hard to play measure 79 so the break between the viola and the second violin isn't clearly audible, like a suture that has been sewn together and left to heal. Measures 85–88 contain extreme contrasts of register that must have perplexed Beethoven's first hearers, who were unaccustomed to hearing a string quartet divided this way.

The experience of listening to this music in 1807—which is when the first performances took place—must have been like walking down a familiar city street and hearing sounds that did not seem to belong there because they had never been heard before. This is something that would happen repeatedly to European city dwellers in the course of the nineteenth century as the Industrial Revolution dramatically transformed the urban landscape and soundscape, and each generation grew accustomed to sights and sounds that would have baffled their predecessors. They were thus challenged on a regular basis to connect what they heard with what they saw, since neither could be assumed to follow traditional rules.[12] The same was true in music, and Beethoven's later works increasingly led listeners to blur the boundaries between aural and visual imagery. An observer at an early performance of Beethoven's Ninth Symphony in 1825 described what he heard this way:

> If at first hearing much seems baroque and strange to the unbiased listener, the eye is nevertheless struck soon and often enough by the lightning bolts that Beethoven's spirit lets loose throughout. This applies particularly to the first Allegro and the Adagio. The former begins with a tremolo in the string instruments, out of which individual wind instruments gradually emerge, like foggy forms from the calm sea, and then at once becomes powerful and grandiose with a series of self-sufficient chords.[13]

Note the extremely visual nature of this description. It is the eye, not the ear, that is struck by the unfolding scene. Lightning bolts emerge from a dark sky; images arise out of the fog and the sea. Another commenter on the same performance, which took place at the Lower Rhine Music Festival in Aachen, wrote that in the instrumental movements "it seems to us that the master wanted to portray . . . confusion, the driving and urgency of great crowds—for example at a folk festival—in which at times a powerful voice asserts itself here and there, but soon sinks in the confusion, in the giddiness and wild jubilation, until the singer finally succeeds in stilling the tumult."[14] Here the appeal is to a voice that stills the crowd, but the prevailing metaphor is still one of confusion imagined in visual terms: the crowds rushing around wildly, the singer imposing order on the chaos. Both writers found the music baffling, its content unclear, but both were willing to venture interpretations of what the strange sounds might look like. Both offered a visual scene to help interpret the unfamiliar auditory scene.

This kind of writing about Beethoven was not uncommon in the 1820s. Adolf Bernhard Marx, one of the most influential critics and pedagogues of his time, thought that "the ability to 'hear' the visual and psychological images suggested by music was the mark of a sophisticated listener in step with his time."[15] Marx was very deliberate in naming Beethoven as the composer who had made this possible. Writing in 1827 about Beethoven's incidental music to Goethe's *Egmont*, Op. 84, he identified it as "the first [composition] in which instrumental music was consciously and intentionally used for the self-sufficient representation of an idea and of actions in progress. . . . Naturally," Marx wrote, "those innumerable artists and dilettantes for whom music remains in the ear, and who hear only sounds, have not been able to accompany him in this direction." Marx then identified the eighteen-year-old Felix Mendelssohn as the only composer who had been able to imitate Beethoven in this regard. Marx cited Mendelssohn's overture to *A Midsummer Night's Dream* but also his early Piano Sonata in E major, op. 6, which had no program or story but which clearly imitated aspects of Beethoven's late style; its episodic construction is sufficiently confusing that it virtually demands extramusical interpretation.[16] Like Beethoven, Mendelssohn was inviting the listener to see his music as well as hear it, or so Marx would have us believe.

It may not be immediately clear why Marx considered this a novelty. Composers throughout the eighteenth century had used music to evoke visual images; one need only think of Vivaldi's *Four Seasons* or Haydn's *Creation*. Such music, though, was self-explanatory. Descriptive pieces came with titles that told listeners what to hear and performers what to imitate. Beethoven was following in a long tradition when he evoked the calls of the nightingale, the quail, and the cuckoo in the second movement of the *Pastoral* Symphony or painted a musical thunderstorm in the fourth movement.

Marx and the anonymous writers quoted above, on the other

hand, were describing music whose pictorial associations were less obvious. The images they evoked were esoteric, and hearing them required imagination and careful listening. The search for such images in Beethoven's music may very well have been inspired by one of the most familiar descriptions of that music ever written: E. T. A. Hoffmann's review of the Fifth Symphony, first published in the *Allgemeine musikalische Zeitung* in 1810 and quoted and paraphrased countless times by others in the ensuing decades. Instrumental music, Hoffmann had written, "disdaining all help, all admixture of any other art, purely expresses the peculiar essence of this art, which can be recognized in it alone."[17] Composers who had tried to paint pictures and events with music, Hoffmann said, were ludicrously mistaken. And then, strangely, he gave a deeply visual description of the experience of listening to Beethoven's instrumental music, which "opens up to us the kingdom of the gigantic and the immeasurable. Glowing beams shoot through this kingdom's deep night, and we become aware of gigantic shadows that surge up and down, enclosing us more and more narrowly and annihilating everything within us."[18]

Deirdre Loughridge has recently offered some valuable perspectives on Hoffmann's review that help explain what he was doing and why.

The review is suffused with ghostly imagery—specifically the idea of "shadows that ... draw closer and closer in upon us"—that conjures the phantasmagoria, a contemporary form of public entertainment in which a hidden image-projection apparatus made approaching ghosts seem terrifyingly real. ... The review thus suggests "seeing" Beethoven's crescendo [in the transition to the fourth movement] as a ghostly shadow emerging from a great distance and finally looming toward one, the hushed opening indicating remoteness, the growing volume and registral spread increasing proximity. The effect relies not on a representation of light in sound but on an analogous technique for creating the illusion of three-dimensional motion in space, and with it a heightened sense of immersion in another world.[19]

Beethoven, in other words, was providing a musical analogue for a sophisticated technological trick meant to mystify and delight its audiences. Most of those who saw the phantasmagoria had no idea how the illusion was created and were thus all the more taken with it. By the same token, those who heard Beethoven's Fifth Symphony were mystified and overwhelmed, but this allowed the music to make them, in Hoffmann's words, *entzückte Geisterseher*: enchanted spirit-seers.[20] Listening to Beethoven, people could see, with their mind's eye, things that their rational minds told them were not real. This music wasn't painting images; it was creating them.[21]

Hoffmann was not satisfied with simply pointing this out, though. He also opened the stage door and invited his audiences to see the machinery that was making the illusion possible. He started by quoting the first twenty-one measures of the symphony in full score: an extravagance even today, and all the more at a time when score publications were rare. His readers could immediately begin to see that, as Hoffmann would state a few pages later, "there is no simpler idea than that which the master laid as the foundation of this entire Allegro and one realizes with wonder how he was able to align all the secondary ideas, all the transitional passages with the rhythmic content of this simple theme in such a way that they served continually to unfold the character of the whole, which that theme could only suggest."[22] Hoffmann spent much of the rest of the review elaborating on this point with technical descriptions of the score, but the extensive examples of printed music he included throughout helped to reinforce it as well. To understand this music, he showed his readers, it was necessary to look at it in detail. Then you could begin to see things that were not at first evident and to grasp the artistry with which Beethoven had put the Fifth Symphony together. Since symphonies before this time had hardly ever been published in score, Hoffmann was showing his readers something they might not have previously imagined being able to see. But his review, like the ones cited earlier, shows the extent to which Beethoven's increasing focus on music's visual dimensions affected others as well; it encouraged them to see things in the music that they would not otherwise have imagined. All of these critics wanted to make sure their readers could see what they were seeing.

Hoffmann was not unique in challenging his readers to see what Beethoven was doing; similar extended commentaries appeared after the Third, Sixth, Seventh, and Eighth Symphonies were published, all rife with printed examples.[23] While it was not unusual for the music journals of the time to include some snippets of music for readers to examine, these reviews go into such detail about the music's unfolding structure, and include so many printed notes, that they risk appearing tedious. But the authors' goal is precisely to bring the profusion of details in Beethoven's music to the attention of the reader's eyes.

Like Hoffmann, they often made connections from the written notes to visual experiences. This was particularly true of the early reviewers of the Ninth Symphony and other late works. As Joseph Fröhlich wrote in 1828 after studying the Ninth extensively,

the deeper were the outlines with which the great master indicated each individual part and displayed it full of life through glowing colors, the more these were brought to the fore by the stark contrasts inherent in them, the more

these individual pictures joined together in his contempla-
tion into a whole through continuous, diligent study, the
clearer did it become . . . that Beethoven did not wish to
write here a symphony of the customary kind . . . that he
was aiming for something extraordinary, completely new.[24]

Fröhlich apparently had an orchestra at his disposal to assist
him in making sense of the way the symphony sounded, but
his language was primarily visual: the music had outlines, colors, and individual pictures joined into a whole. The result was
music that asked not just to be heard but to be envisioned, in
this case as a grand, interconnected tapestry. What was de-
picted, Fröhlich suggested, was the composer's autobiography
in tones—a novel idea at the time but one that has since been
widely applied to much of Beethoven's other music as well, as
we saw in chapter 3.

Later the same year, Friedrich Rochlitz, struggling to make
sense of the Quartet in C-sharp minor, op. 131, described in the
third person the following experience with this novel and unusual work.

He had first received it engraved in parts. . . . Not unaccustomed to occupying himself with music . . . in such
pieces, he spread the parts out next to one another, certainly not hoping thereby to become exactly familiar with
the work—to master it—but rather to instruct himself
about its essence, its purpose, its construction and its manner, and thereby to enjoy an agreeable first course. He had
expected something unusual, indeed strange, but what he
now found appeared so motley and irregular, at times so
highly singular and arbitrary, that he often did not know
what to make of it. The melodies—what could be dis-
cerned of them in such isolation—for the most part com-

pletely odd, but deeply gripping, even, perhaps, incisive . . . The modulations not infrequently pushed to the point of being bizarre, indeed grating. And so, in every aspect, including outward arrangement (like an overly large fantasy, ever changing and transforming anew), the key (C-sharp minor, predominantly, but in its course pretty much all keys in the chromatic scale more or less touched upon) and the time signatures (in the most singular succession, always interrupting one another, from the simplest to the most artificial, for example nine-four meter), almost everything . . . appeared to him motley and irregular, much most singular, much entirely arbitrary. Out of all of it, what became truly clear to him and spoke to his heart was so little that he could not put it into words. He believed only that he could surmise more than he understood, that the deep shaft, so troublesome to traverse, was as rich in veins of gold as any that Beethoven had discovered and excavated.[25]

The experience Rochlitz described was nearly unprecedented. His protagonist—he claimed to be describing the experience of a friend—received the music in parts, which is how chamber music at the time was normally printed. Determined to try to make sense of this unusual work—it is in seven movements, played without break—he laid out the parts and tried to make them cohere visually. What he saw he compared to a mine, and the details that stood out to veins of gold. The language in which Rochlitz cast this experience suggests that Beethoven had already dug out the ore but that it remained for listeners and performers to refine it, perhaps in part by completing the visual imagery that Rochlitz's friend could only surmise.

As these examples make clear, esoteric visual scenes were common currency among those struggling to make sense of

Beethoven's most challenging music. When something didn't seem musically coherent, the instinctive reaction was to appeal to the eyes to explain it, not as program music but as something much more novel and ingenious. This could be done either by evoking extramusical imagery or by describing how the music looked on paper, appealing to the listener to "see for yourself." Hoffmann and the other critics just cited did both, often in the same breath.

What they were seeing can be illuminated by once again looking at what Beethoven saw, this time while writing one of his most vigorously rhythmic works: the Seventh Symphony. This is the piece he was sketching in 1811 when he complained, on an adjacent page, about the intolerable noises in his ears. Wagner called the Seventh Symphony "the apotheosis of the dance ... the happiest realization of the movements of the body in an ideal form,"[26] giving voice to the commonly shared intuition that this is an intensely physical work. The *Vivace* section of the first movement is dominated by a distinctive rhythm consisting of a dotted eighth note followed by a sixteenth note and an eighth note in 6/8 time. It is notoriously difficult to play this rhythm repeatedly and accurately, but when a conductor and orchestra get into the groove—as exemplified, perhaps, in Toscanini's 1936 recording with the New York Philharmonic— the result is viscerally thrilling. This is certainly a piece that shows it is not enough just to hear music; both performers and listeners are called to embody it, with all the senses at their disposal. It is hardly surprising that a composer with progressive hearing loss would be drawn to create music like this.

Beethoven even seems to have gotten into the groove while sketching this symphony. It was at the beginning of the Petter sketchbook, in which he worked extensively on the Seventh Symphony, that Beethoven complained about the noise in his ears when he worked at the piano. Later in the sketchbook

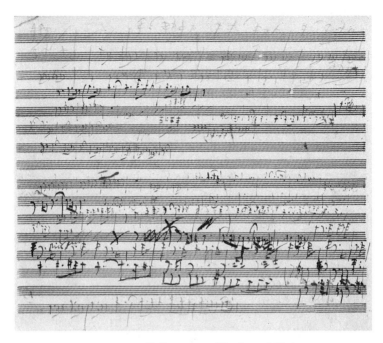

FIGURE 14. Folio 11 recto of Beethoven's Petter
sketchbook, showing sketches for the first movement
of the Seventh Symphony. From the collection of the
Beethoven-Haus in Bonn. Used by permission.

he seems to have broken free. Page after page is occupied by
seemingly chaotic notations centering on the single distinctive
rhythmic pattern of the symphony's first movement. Folio 11
recto (fig. 14) can serve as an example; it contains both pencil
and ink notations that fill up nearly all the space available on the
page's sixteen staves and some of the space in between as well.
As with the examples discussed earlier in this chapter, the very
appearance of these hard-to-decipher, single-line scrawls —
seemingly so different from the more orderly finished score —
tells us something of great importance. In writing them, Beethoven did the same thing over and over; he drew the three
notes in quick vertical motions, then wrote the beam that connects them, the shorter beam that makes the second note into

a sixteenth, and finally the dot after the first note. Three quick
vertical motions, progressing from left to right, are followed by
three even quicker horizontal ones—Beethoven's haste can be
judged from the fact that these thick lines across the page often fall short of the necessary length; the beam at the bottom
may not reach the third note of the triplet, and the sixteenth-
note beam may not quite connect. The result has the look of
Chinese calligraphy, with carefully learned pen strokes tossed
off in great haste. Perhaps it also brings to mind early chant
notation, in which complex neumes signifying collections of
pitches were written without staff lines, their elegant shape
embodying the curves of melodies that were already known by
heart. There is no question that Beethoven felt a rhythm as he
sketched. It is a different rhythm from that conveyed in the music, but he must have been physically obsessed with writing it
in the same way he expected his players to be obsessed with its
performance. The anonymous writer quoted in the last chapter
recalls how Beethoven carefully followed Schuppanzigh's bowing during the first performance of the Seventh Symphony and
beat time accordingly. Both writing and performing this music,
he depended on his eyes. But he also depended on something
more: the convergence of seeing with physical experience—
the feel of the pen strokes on the paper, the synchrony with his
first violinist in marking time. Even Spohr's mocking account
of Beethoven conducting this symphony points up the intense
physicality of the music for the composer: something the old-
fashioned Spohr, accustomed to greater decorum, could only
see as mildly ridiculous.

As with so much of Beethoven's other music, this symphony
would also be interpreted by his contemporaries as a visual
scene. With growing awareness of Beethoven's deafness during
the 1820s, together with the increasing prominence during the
1820s of visual descriptions like those quoted in this chapter,
the connection between the aural and the visual in Beetho-

ven became almost a cliché, causing some writers to indulge in flights of imagination at which more sober modern readers can only roll their eyes. Writing in 1825, Carl Friedrich Ebers described the entire symphony as a depiction of a wedding.

> In the Poco sostenuto the double doors of the great hall are opened; the climbing basses and violins, from the tenth measure on, are old, stiff men and women of the family, who walk about in the hall and arrange things in various ways. At the Vivace, the guests now gradually appear. Various characters, steady, lightfooted, comical and sentimental figures are united in the formation of a whole, which, however, stands forth only as a bright mix of colors.[27]

Then, in the last movement,

> propriety is no longer heeded, the spirit of wine shows itself everywhere. As often happens at weddings, baptisms, and balls of this kind, bickering arises. . . . People become wanton, destroying tables, mirrors, chandeliers; the inevitable consequences of overindulgence show themselves, which the basses seem to indicate clearly. In short, the whole ends with a general confusion, where only a few triumphantly hold their ground.[28]

All of this was submitted by Ebers in response to the question "What do you find in this tone-painting [*Tongemälde*]?" These comments by one of the day's leading composers were given prominent space in one of the leading music journals of the day, suggesting that they were taken quite seriously by musicians and readers alike. "Tone-painting" had indeed become a major theme in the interpretation of Beethoven's music.

Two centuries later, the visual images that Beethoven's contemporaries discovered in his music with such excitement may no longer occur to us or move us in the same way. At a time when popular music is increasingly being enhanced by state-of-the-art visual technology, our experience of classical music has become formal and rigid. It is hard to understand what Hoffmann, Fröhlich, and the other writers just cited were getting at, so we often tend to dismiss what they had to say with a smirk of condescension. What I hope to suggest in the epilogue is that the way they heard Beethoven's music reflects an understanding of its wholeness—of human wholeness—that we would do well to seek to recover. Here Beethoven's and Barbara's stories intersect once again, in a way that has to do with far more than just the shared experience of deafness.

Embracing Wholeness

In the summer of 2008 I went to a water park in Texas with Barbara and our two children, then sixteen and fourteen years old. She and I made an odd pair. For safety's sake I had to leave my glasses in a locker, and Barbara had to leave her "ears." Profoundly nearsighted, I let my profoundly deaf wife lead me around while she relied on me for auditory information. Together the four of us climbed stairs and slid down chutes, cavorted around the lazy river wrapped in inner tubes, and lounged in the pool.

Our first visit to the park the day before had not been so successful. Barbara had drifted ahead of us on the lazy river and gotten separated from us. Unable to hear, she had been led to an office by the staff and kept uninformed for two or three hours until I was finally able to locate her. The incident is reminiscent of a story about how Beethoven, walking through the countryside in his last years, was arrested as a vagrant, due to his unkempt appearance, and held against his will until a prominent musician could identify him.[1] The fact that both he and Barbara could speak, read, and write seemed not to matter; Beethoven was not believed, and Barbara was given meaningless assurances while being repeatedly ignored, even though I had spoken to the security staff and asked them to keep a watch out for my deaf wife. We can imagine that Beethoven and Barbara felt much the same way: panicked, frustrated, and deeply alone. Then as now, society does not have a good grasp of how to relate to a lone and isolated deaf person.

For our family, this was just one confusing incident among many. What makes it memorable is that we returned and redeemed the experience the next day. We were determined to have fun and to enjoy time together, and with some persistence we pulled it off. Barbara did not transcend or overcome her deafness, any more than I transcended or overcame my nearsightedness. Rather, we lent each other support and embraced a kind of wholeness that thrives in spite of human fragility.

There were many other such moments of paradoxical wholeness as Barbara's health continued to decline. On a trip to Enchanted Rock, a popular natural attraction in Texas, she climbed with me as far as she could make it before her lack of balance forced her to stop; I walked a bit farther before returning to help her back down. We did make it to Laurel Falls in the Smoky Mountains with extended family; this easy hike was as much as she could tolerate, and that only by gritting her teeth and pushing on when all her instincts told her to stop. On reaching the falls she broke down and wept, releasing the panic she had pushed aside during the ascent, then sat down with us to eat a picnic lunch and finally enjoy the scene. Ominous thunder rolled in the background, but the storm never broke upon us; it was simply a coda to the wide-ranging symphony of emotions we had just witnessed.

In the fall of 2011 Barbara and I took a memorable trip to California, where she heard me deliver a paper at a conference for the first time, sitting in the first row and following along in a written copy I had given her. She leaned on my arm to keep from falling as we negotiated the hills of San Francisco, climbing to Ghirardelli Square for dessert after a seafood dinner at

Fisherman's Wharf. All of these achievements were small triumphs at best, but they all required cooperation, accommodation, patience, and humility. By supporting each other, we discovered and reinforced those qualities in ourselves—qualities that had always been there but that we learned to use in powerful new ways.

There were also moments when deafness and its consequences overwhelmed both of our defenses. For Barbara, facing a sudden loss of hearing was the most challenging experience of her life, far more challenging than her cancer. Even secondhand, I felt the isolation she experienced and shared in it. During our first months in Waco, before Barbara got the first implant, my whole life was devoted to beginning my new job and being present for my family. There was no time, and precious little energy, left to make social connections and truly join the community to which I had moved. The things I was experiencing were impossible to talk about with others, who were simply unable to imagine what it was like to be in my position. For the first time in decades, depression threatened to overwhelm my defenses, and I took medication to deal with its effects. Barbara took it as well, because whatever I experienced, she experienced ten times over, and she struggled in ways even I could not grasp. She would take antidepressants for the rest of her life, and the wholeness she and I found was thus supported by yet another medical miracle that was not available to Beethoven.

Beethoven's own struggles with depression are something we have repeatedly had occasion to observe, and they are easy to understand. Before he left for Vienna in 1792, Count Waldstein famously told him, "With the help of assiduous labor you shall receive Mozart's spirit from Haydn's hands." Mozart's genius, Waldstein wrote, was mourning the death of her pupil and wished to form a union with another. Noting this, Thayer observed, "It proves how great were the writer's hopes, how strong his faith in Beethoven."[2]

But it proves something else as well. At the age of twenty-one, Beethoven was being saddled with an expectation he could not reasonably hope to fulfill. Of course the expression was metaphorical, and Waldstein intended to offer encouragement, not an unattainable goal. Nevertheless his choice of words is telling. Like Alice Miller's prototypical gifted child described in chapter 1, Beethoven had become accustomed to extravagant praise for his talents and achievements. Waldstein thought it was perfectly reasonable to expect him to become a second Mozart, and Beethoven may well have agreed. Miller's description, though, makes it understandable that he was also haunted by depression, which came to the fore when circumstances denied him the easy fix of professional success. Deafness was thus more than just a musical crisis for Beethoven. From its first appearance, it threatened to draw back the curtain and reveal the emptiness behind the persona he had been forced to construct during his difficult childhood.

In order to fully understand Beethoven's deafness, therefore, it is necessary to seek to understand his depression as well. As we saw in chapter 1, that depression, so vivid at the time of the Heiligenstadt crisis, returned in the mid-1810s when Beethoven was at the peak of his public success but his hearing was entering its final decline. As it was for Barbara and me, finding a way through and beyond depression was part of the wholeness that Beethoven achieved: a wholeness that required descending into the deepest and most bleakly forbidding corners of his soul so that new things might grow in the hostile terrain he found there.

The experience of clinical depression has been described by gifted writers throughout history: for the modern era perhaps most definitively by Dante, who spoke of finding himself in a dark forest in the midst of life's journey, a forest so savage and bitter that merely to think about it was to experience its terror anew. Dante persisted in order to tell of the good he found there, and proceeded to describe a journey into hell followed by an ascent to greater knowledge and understanding. Of those who have chronicled that journey more recently, few have been more eloquent than Parker Palmer, who wrote of his own depression as part of the process of discovering his vocation. He recalled a breakthrough when a therapist said, "You seem to look upon depression as the hand of an enemy trying to crush you. Do you think you could see it instead as the hand of a friend, pressing you down onto ground on which it is safe to stand?"[3] Palmer spoke of this experience in great depth in an interview for public radio, in which he explained that a heart broken by depression acquires a "greater capacity to hold the whole range of human experience. . . . I think it's possible to grow a larger heart that is able to hold what life gives it."[4]

Depression, as Beethoven described it at Heiligenstadt, is a deadening of emotional range, a flattening out into the ground. What Palmer suggests is that to recover from depression is to gain an expanded capacity to feel the full reach of human emotion: both grief and joy in greater measure, as well as the range of nuanced feelings in between and around them. This is perhaps what E. T. A. Hoffmann meant when he spoke, in his review of Beethoven's Fifth Symphony, of "this pain, which, consuming love, hope, and joy within itself, seeks to burst our breast asunder with a full-voiced consonance of all the passions," or when he compared Beethoven's and Shakespeare's work to "a lovely tree, whose buds and leaves, flowers and fruits all grow from the same seed" despite an apparent lack of unity.[5]

For Beethoven, depression was closely linked to deafness; deafness was the source of his depression at Heiligenstadt and again in the mid-1810s, and probably at other times as well. Furthermore, the metaphor of flattening could be used to describe both deafness and depression, albeit in different ways. Deafness flattened his experience of music, causing him to broaden it in directions that would otherwise not have occurred to him. Depression flattened his emotional life, but he responded by broadening the expressive range of the music he was writing. As his deafness grew, his music became more tactile, more visual, and more emotionally dynamic, revealing in all three of these dimensions essential aspects of the art that previous composers, not flattened as he was, had not pursued to quite the same extremes.

At the same time, like Barbara, Beethoven grew a larger heart that was able to hold what life put into it. For those who knew Barbara, this was evident in her calm stoicism, in the intensity of her everyday joy, and in the strength of her grieving as well: grieving for her first husband and child, grieving for her lost health and then for her lost hearing, grieving for the life she and I had enjoyed before her deafness and would never have again. For those who know Beethoven's music, it is evident in the tragic defiance and triumph of the Fifth Symphony but also in the relaxed humor of the Eighth; in the lyricism of the *Archduke* Trio and the ecstatic mysticism of the *Missa Solemnis*; in the frivolity of the G Major String Quartet, op. 18, no. 2, as well as in the expansive breadth of the "Razumovsky" quartets, op. 59. Whatever they may express individually, Beethoven's works, taken together, illustrate the emotional complexity of a fully realized human life. His deafness and depression helped make the high points higher and the low points lower, but he remained the same person throughout. If we are to remythologize his music for our times, it should be as a paragon of wholeness, and hence, paradoxically, of health: the health that belongs not to a perfectly functioning body but to a vital and unified spirit.

This kind of health avoids both the heroic and the tragic stereotypes that are often applied to Beethoven's life and music and offers something both desirable and attainable to the rest of us: those who, like Barbara, live their lives as honestly as possible in the face of adversity, capitalizing on what is offered to them while making their peace with what is not. Hearing Beethoven through Barbara's ears, we can see that his example is more humane than heroic, more typical than tragic. The spiritual growth his music traces is not that of a lone figure reaching heights others cannot share. Deafness gave him the chance to become more fully human, more universal, and to remind the modern world of how music can serve both of those ends.

December 16, 1826, was Beethoven's fifty-sixth, and last, birthday. On December 19, 2011, my own fifty-sixth birthday, Barbara and I were preparing to go out to celebrate when she began feeling dizzy and feverish. Her condition became alarming enough that I hurried her into the car, still dressed for dinner, and took her to the emergency room. By the time we got there she needed a wheelchair, and when we finally reached a patient room she had a violent headache and her tongue and the back of her mouth were becoming numb. Because lack of sensation in her throat might cause her to suffocate on aspirated fluids, she was quickly placed under anesthesia. I never spoke to her again.

After her final CT scan, which showed that massive bleeding was choking her brainstem—unstoppable because of the blood thinners she was taking to prevent another stroke—she was moved to the ICU. She remained there for three days on life support until a transplant crew could be flown in to attempt to harvest her organs. This they did in the wee hours of Friday, December 23. Her kidneys were no longer usable, but her corneas, soft tissue, and sections of bone may have helped dozens of others to see, recover from burns, and undergo complex orthopedic surgery. We buried Barbara two days after Christmas. Less than three months short of her own fifty-sixth birthday, her charmed, vexed, miraculous, improbable life had finally run out. The neurosurgeon on duty that night told me he had never heard of a patient with an astrocytoma—that particular kind of brain tumor—who had survived for as long as she had, with comparable quality of life.

Barbara was often deeply unhappy with the way things had turned out for her. While she rarely complained in public, I knew how great her struggle was. At the same time, she enjoyed her life, treasured me and the children, and was grateful for each small, incremental improvement in her condition. She made a fragile peace with the way she lived that enabled her to withstand disappointments and challenges that could seem overwhelming. She did not overcome those challenges; she found wholeness by learning to live within them.

This reality of Barbara's life was evident to those of us who knew her best. Others may have seen her as a survivor, as a tough lady who handled everything life threw at her with grace, while to some she probably seemed an unfortunate who never had a fair chance. In truth she was zesty, fun-loving, painfully shy, inhibited, generous, and sometimes resentful. She believed deeply in God, with "the faith of a child," but she was baffled by injustice, particularly her own. She was ambushed regularly by painful memories, but she could just as easily be happy settling next to me for a drive to the grocery store, and she felt passionate enthusiasm for the places and experiences that had enriched her early life: camping in Yosemite as a child, singing Handel's *Messiah* in college and afterward, decorating the house and baking cookies and other confections for Christmas. Barbara was a whole person, and the simple joy she could bring to unbearable circumstances made it all the harder to see the deep pain to which those same circumstances could and did reduce her. In popular parlance it would be fair to call her a hero, a saint, or a martyr, but much of her life was anything but heroic, and neither sainthood nor martyrdom gave her much satisfaction when she merely longed to be herself.

Barbara's wholeness transcended chronology. After deafness she was still the same person she had been before: indeed, she was the same person she had been before cancer. She allowed herself to be identified as a cancer survivor, but she didn't embrace the identity, any more than she embraced being deaf. She didn't want either of those conditions to define her.

We see a similar kind of wholeness in Beethoven's life. Before his hearing failed he was already giving unprecedented attention to the writing process and responding creatively to the feel and touch of the pianos at his disposal. Afterward he continued to do these things, although he took them in different directions than he might have had his hearing remained intact, and he wrote different music as a result. His life and his music nevertheless remained whole: single entities touched but not defined by deafness. Beethoven did not overcome deafness; he found himself through and along with it.

The myths that have defined our understanding of Beethoven are painted with a broad brush, and they do not serve this reality well. He has often been portrayed as a mighty force of nature, a hero who defied fate and triumphed over adversity. Scott Burnham rightly refers to the Beethoven of popular understanding as a "demigod."[6] This Beethoven speaks in absolutes: fate can be overcome, the power of the human spirit knows no limits. A handful of works is often brought forward to support this view, and they have been given disproportionate attention. The *Eroica* Symphony, for example, has been taken as emblematic of Beethoven's entire middle period, extending from the time it was written until the Congress of Vienna; this is now commonly known as Beethoven's "heroic period."

But to hear only triumph and heroism in Beethoven's music is to miss its full emotional range, which extends to tragedy, lyricism, vulnerability, and fragility as well, sometimes within one and the same piece. Like Barbara, Beethoven found wholeness by embracing the entirety of life, finding new resources within himself even while accepting the limitations that were dealt him.

If there is one thing that looking closely at his deafness and his response to it makes clear, it is that the materials he used were chosen for practical reasons, not as means to an end. He relied extensively on writing because the written page was congenial to him and increasingly necessary as his hearing grew worse. He created new musical textures with his eyes because it came more naturally than depending on his failing ears. He made unprecedented use of short, memorable fragments because these fit easily into his mental Rolodex. He created long, complex musical structures because these could be planned visually, with the fragments serving as bricks and mortar to fill in the frame. The results were often highly rhythmic, as, in their own way, were the sketches and manuscripts from which they sprang. Even his relationship with his pianos grew in tandem with his deafness, his physical bond with the instrument becoming palpable in his late sonatas, bagatelles, and variations.

Here, though, one must look for the small effect rather than the long-range structure. The bagatelles of Opus 126, for example—virtually his last completed works for piano—contain passages seemingly designed to get the Broadwood's frame vibrating by linking an oscillating bass with right-hand melodies that reinforce the harmonics from the opposite end of the keyboard. This happens notably when Beethoven uses an exaggerated *musette* texture to imitate the sound of the bagpipe in the middle section of No. 4 in B Minor (example 8.1), while No. 6 in E-flat Major has nearly twelve measures of a fast, rocking open fifth

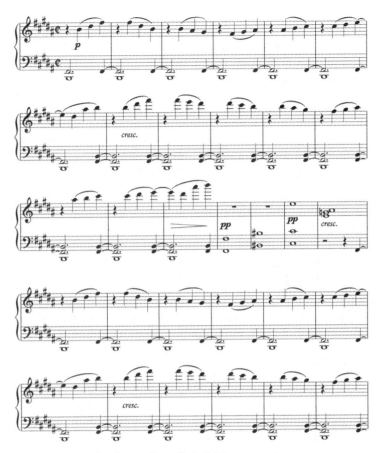

EXAMPLE 8.1. Beethoven, Bagatelle in B Minor, op. 126, no. 4, mm. 52–105

in the left hand, over which the right hand rises in ascending thirds to a peak four and a half octaves above the bass (example 8.2). Moments like this show Beethoven listening to his instrument with his body, responding as much to touch as to actual sound. In this sense they resemble the portions of Opus 109 and 110 discussed in chapter 5, except that they never rise much above the dynamic level of *piano*. By 1824, when these pieces were written, the increasingly deaf Beethoven must have understood that more volume was not necessarily needed

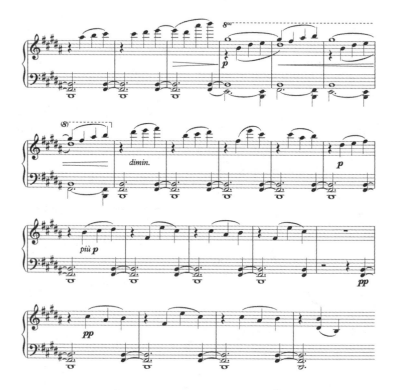

to make the music physically palpable. The feeling of his fingers gently undulating across the Broadwood's deep keys was sufficient.[7]

If we are looking for "Beethoven," then, we must not limit ourselves to what is loud, long, or extensively worked out. His response to his deafness led him in the other direction as well. In either case — whether he was seeking to "have the whole in view" while creating a huge work like the *Eroica* or to coax a physical connection from his piano as in the late bagatelles — changing music cannot have been his goal. The truths he revealed were true already: that music engages sight and touch as well as hearing; that it originates in the body; that it is definitively shaped by the physical materials of its creation. Beethoven

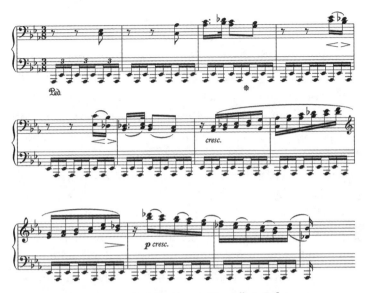

EXAMPLE 8.2. Beethoven, Bagatelle in E-flat
Major, op. 126, no. 6, mm. 33–44

got a bit closer to music in its wholeness because he had to labor under what many perceive as a limitation. In doing so he discovered things about music that had always been true, but that deafness allowed him to demonstrate in unique ways.

Musical wholeness, emotional wholeness: both spring from the same source. If Beethoven revealed new dimensions of music, it should not be surprising that he expanded music's expressive vocabulary as well. If anything, deafness was even more central to this aspect of his creative life than it was to the technical ones just mentioned, because it forced him to explore new dimensions not just in music but in himself.

The wholeness of Beethoven's music is especially easy to see if we view Beethoven's oeuvre as a single sustained musical record of a life that began in Bonn and continued to evolve through growing deafness and beyond. Throughout that life Beethoven sought wholeness because it eluded him, as it was bound to do given the expectations that were laid out for him as a child and a young adult.

Neither Beethoven nor Barbara would have chosen the paths their lives followed, but both walked those paths in full view of others, stumbled at times, and persisted, led by the gifts they were given and the vocation they sought. Both, therefore, gifted others with an example that cajoles but does not coerce. The emotional highs of Beethoven's music—the familiar passages of overwhelming tragedy and triumph—are a part of the example he set, but they were never meant to stand on their own. The joviality, the lyricism, the whimsy, the sometimes startling juxtapositions—these are all part of the package as well. Stricken by deafness, Barbara found a life she did not expect but that transformed her, our family, and everyone who opened their hearts to us. Beethoven, facing the same affliction, nevertheless found a music that would let all the fullness of human life resound.

Acknowledgments

Without Barbara, there would have been no book. This is, first and foremost, an expression of my respect and admiration for the strongest and most courageous person I have ever known. Thank you, my love, for everything.

A little over a year after Barbara's death, I began dating my present wife, Meg, a freelance editor and indexer in Chicago whom I knew through mutual friends. Early in 2014 we were married, although circumstances compelled us to live nine hundred miles apart until mid-2015, when a yearlong sabbatical from Baylor allowed me both to write this book and to move to Chicago for a year to be with Meg. As I completed the book in the summer of 2016, Meg was finally able to join me back in Waco, where she is happily beginning a new career in midlife.

Although it's not entirely clear to either of us how it happened, the conception of this book took place during the two-city phase, when we could see each other only for short times and the exchange of intellectual ideas flowed like a torrent. All I can say for sure is that it was my idea to use my experience with Barbara's deafness to gain insight into Beethoven's music, and that Meg kept returning to the example of Simon Winchester's *The Professor and the Madman*, which combines two very different life stories into a compelling narrative that also describes one of the great intellectual achievements of modern times: the creation of the *Oxford English Dictionary*. If I have done something even remotely comparable in these pages, it is thanks to Meg's patient support, insight, and deep knowledge of how books are crafted. I have been very fortunate in my partners in life.

The shape of the book was also transformed by an extraordinary instance of serendipity. In the fall of 2014, Tom Beghin visited Baylor to present a lecture. A colleague asked me to pick him up at the airport, and although we had never met before, we immediately began talking about Beethoven, deafness, pianos, and the seemingly impractical idea of trying to re-create the resonator that Beethoven used during his final years to try to hear his instrument better. The conversation continued through emails and Skype chats, and less than two years later I was in Belgium, in the workshop of master piano craftsman Chris Maene, examining Maene's re-creation of Beethoven's Broadwood and the first stages of acoustician Thomas Wulfrank's reconstruction of what they had come to call "the hearing machine." Their work was based on scrupulous study of the discussions of the project in Beethoven's conversation books, conducted by Tom, Tilman Skowroneck, and others. As it turns out, *Inside the Hearing Machine*, Tom's recording of the last three Beethoven sonatas using an acoustically optimized version of the resonator, will be released before this book goes to press. I think it is fair to say, though, that neither would have emerged in anything like its present form without the other. I owe Tom, Tilman, and the entire crew at the Orpheus Institute in Ghent a resounding round of thanks. Scholarship and music making have rarely harmonized so thoroughly and with such intriguing results.

Also coincidentally, the American Musicological Society's annual meeting in Louisville, Kentucky, in 2015 featured a panel on "music and deafness." This brought me into contact with other scholars who were studying the same issue, and I learned an enormous amount from them while also gaining confidence from their support for and interest in my project. I must particularly thank Jeannette Jones, with whom I copresented a paper at the next year's AMS meeting in Vancouver on a panel sponsored by the Society's Study Group on Music and Disability, along with Jessica Holmes and Andrew Dell'Antonio, who provided their own valuable contributions and insights. The entire disability studies community—too many to name—has helped sensitize me to the perfectly reasonable desire of disabled people to be treated like everybody else, as fully human, and to the various ways in which how we speak and write about disability can detract from or contribute to that goal. If my own human failings have occasionally caused me to fall short while discussing this complex topic, I take full responsibility.

During my time in Chicago, the libraries at Northwestern University granted me full access and checkout privileges, allowing me to use them as my home base. I am also grateful to the staff of Northwestern's Auditory Neuroscience Laboratory, especially Joan Hargrave, Nina Kraus, Jessica MacLean, and Trent Nicol, for letting me tour their facilities and pepper them with questions. I soon realized that while much of their research was far too technical and detailed to fit easily into a book like this, they were as interested in hearing about Barbara's and my experiences as I was in hearing about theirs.

Meg and I lived in the northern Chicago neighborhood of Rogers Park, and Lake Michigan became a kind of silent partner in my research as well. During countless walks I got to know its many moods and colors, and strolling frequently to the end of the Pratt Pier, I learned to feel surrounded by the lake first and the city second, while ideas about Beethoven, Barbara, and deafness germinated from its depths.

Special thanks go to those who let me share their personal stories of coping with hearing loss: my former student Zachary Ridgway, my colleague Doris DeLoach, Lindsay Crocker, Kristin Oberle, and other contributors to the Association of Adult Musicians with Hearing Loss blog who generously responded to questions I posted there. Audiologists Marshall Chasin and John Berry graciously shared their thoughts and ideas, and Kate Gfeller provided valuable insights on the functioning of cochlear implants in the understanding of music. I am also indebted to Theodore Albrecht for sharing with me sections of his forthcoming English-language edition of Beethoven's conversation books, and for some valuable exchanges about some of the key players in the conversations recorded there.

In additional to the sabbatical from Baylor, my work on this book was facilitated by a grant from the University Research Committee, which enabled me to travel to Europe and visit the Beethoven-Haus, the Orpheus Institute in Ghent, and Piano's Maene in Ruiselede: a trip which provided the vital connections that made this book come together. Michael Ladenburger, curator of the Beethoven-Haus museum, repeatedly let me try out the replicas of Beethoven's ear trumpets, and librarian Dorethea Geffert was most helpful in accommodating my sometimes surprising requests.

Many at Baylor also lent a hand. I must particularly thank Tim McKinney, acting dean of the School of Music in 2014–15, who enthusiastically supported my sabbatical application. Kenneth Carriveau helped me gain borrowing privileges at Northwestern, and Clayton Crenshaw and the entire staff of the Crouch Fine Arts Library were unfailingly supportive during the time I worked on the book there before and after my year in Chicago. Carrie Drew, the audiologist who first introduced Barbara and me to the pocket talker, obligingly posed for the photograph in figure 1 to demonstrate its use.

Elizabeth Branch Dyson, my acquisitions editor at Chicago, inspired me with her immediate enthusiasm for the project. Her light but consistently perceptive editorial hand was exactly what was needed as I refined my ideas and sought to forge the diverse chapters and multiple threads into a single continuous narrative. Every writer should be blessed with an editor so encouraging and helpful.

I must also give thanks for the vital contributions made by manuscript editor Ruth Goring, designer Matt Avery, production controller Joseph Claude, and promotions manager Levi Stahl.

In this book I have tried to handle the complex challenge of writing about an interdisciplinary topic in an accessible style. In addition to music and the medical study of deafness, the fields on which I have touched include, at a bare minimum, psychology, music perception, disability studies, sound studies, and neuroscience. It is my hope that specialists in each of these areas may feel inspired to expand on the sometimes bare suggestions offered here, proving through their own contributions that there still remain a vast number of new things to be said about Beethoven and his music.

Robin Wallace
Baylor University
August 2017

Notes

INTRODUCTION

1. Karl-Heinz Köhler and Grita Herre, eds., *Ludwig van Beethovens Konversationshefte* (Leipzig: VEB Deutscher Verlag für Musik, 1972–2001), 1:64. Beethoven did discuss the possibility of treatment by galvanism as early as 1801; see George Thomas Ealy, "Of Ear Trumpets and a Resonance Plate: Early Hearing Aids and Beethoven's Hearing Perception," *19th-Century Music* 17/3 (Spring 1994): 264. For an argument that Beethoven later submitted to such treatment, see Wolfram Klinger, "Das Rätsel von Beethovens Gehörleiden," *Bonner Beethoven-Studien* 5 (2006): 135. Klinger points out that Beethoven wrote in April 1823 that he could not have tolerated galvanism earlier, suggesting that by this time he had actually done so.

CHAPTER ONE

1. This phenomenon has been extensively documented and written about. See, for example, Marshall Chasin, ed., *Hearing Loss in Musicians: Prevention and Management* (San Diego: Plural, 2009). As Jessica Holmes points out ("Expert Listening beyond the Limits of Hearing: Music and Deafness," *Journal of the American Musicological Society* 70 (2017): 204–9), hearing loss has been to some extent romanticized among heavy metal and other rock musicians, but it is still highly stigmatized in the classical music world. Recently the Association of Adult Musicians with Hearing Loss has addressed the issue openly; its online and print publications will be cited later in this book.

2. Since this letter does not specify the year when it was written, the date June 29, 1800, was once widely accepted. Wegeler recalled this as the year he received the letter in his *Biographische Notizen* of Beethoven, published in English as *Beethoven Remembered: The Biographical Notes of Franz Wegeler and*

Ferdinand Ries (Arlington, VA: Great Ocean, 1987), which will henceforth be referred to as Wegeler/Ries; and Alfred Kalischer, who edited the earliest collection of Beethoven's letters, accepted this dating. If it were correct, the letter to Carl Amenda cited later in this chapter would have to be dated to 1800 as well. However, Thayer's dating of the letter to 1801 has been generally accepted by later scholars. See Alan Tyson, "Ferdinand Ries (1784–1838): The History of His Contribution to Beethoven Biography," *19th-Century Music* 7/3 (April 1984): 217 for further specifics.

3. Sieghard Brandenburg, ed., *Ludwig van Beethoven: Briefwechsel Gesamtausgabe* (Munich: G. Henle, 1996), 1:79–80 (no. 65). My translation.

4. Brian F. McCabe, in "Beethoven's Deafness," *Annals of Otology, Rhinology and Laryngology* 67/1 (March 1958): 201, disputed whether Beethoven suffered from loudness recruitment, pointing out that he would not have been able to tolerate the volume level involved in playing a concerto with a full orchestra. Elsewhere, though, the fact of recruitment has been widely accepted. This discrepancy may be explained by the fact, noted below, that Beethoven reported putting cotton in his ears while playing the piano to counteract "the disagreeable noise." When he began doing this, and to what extent he did it, is not clear.

5. Alexander Wheelock Thayer, *Thayer's Life of Beethoven*, rev. and ed. Elliott Forbes (Princeton, NJ: Princeton University Press, 1967), 187. This version of Thayer's biography will henceforth be referred to as Thayer-Forbes. The source cited is the Fischoff manuscript, a collection of documents about which, according to Forbes, "Thayer urged caution in its use for establishing biographical fact" (Thayer-Forbes, xiv).

6. Ibid. Forbes apparently added the confirmation from Nikolaus Zmeskall von Domanovecz, also presumably on the basis of the Fischoff manuscript.

7. See Kenneth M. Stevens and William G. Hemingway, "Beethoven's Deafness," *Journal of the American Medical Association* 213/3 (July 20, 1970): 436–37. "Serious effusion in the middle ear occurs in about 5% of adults with typhoid fever and in more than half of children with typhoid fever. The effusion is often not associated with perforation and may lead to later adhesive otitis. . . . Neurosensory loss associated with typhoid fever was not infrequently encountered by the German otologists. Politzer points out that primary nerve degeneration has been reported in people suffering from typhoid fever." Adam Politzer was the author of *Lehrbuch der Ohrenheilkunde für praktische Ärzte und Studierende*, which went through several editions after its publication in 1878–82 and is considered the standard late nineteenth-century textbook on diseases of the ear.

8. Alexander Wheelock Thayer, *The Life of Ludwig van Beethoven*, ed. and

rev. Henry Edward Krehbiel (New York: G. Schirmer, 1921), 1:263–64. This version of Thayer's biography will henceforth be referred to as Thayer-Krehbiel.

9. Although Thayer-Krehbiel says, "That Beethoven really related this strange story cannot be questioned; the word of the venerable Charles Neate to the author is sufficient on that point," Thayer-Forbes omits it.

10. The aria, "O welch ein Leben!," is listed, along with another aria for soprano, as WoO 91 in the Kinsky-Halm Beethoven catalog. It is based on the "Maigesang," op. 52, no. 4, which despite the high opus number was probably written when Beethoven was still in Bonn. The name of the tenor for whom it was written is not specified. The new edition of the catalog gives 1795 as the most likely year of composition. Kurt Dorfmüller, Norbert Gertsch, and Julia Ronge, eds., *Ludwig van Beethoven: Thematisch-bibliographisches Werkverzeichnis* (Munich: G. Henle, 2014), 1:282–87, 2:222–25.

11. Edward Larkin, "Beethoven's Medical History," in Martin Cooper, *Beethoven: The Last Decade: 1817–1827* (London: Oxford University Press, 1970), 448.

12. Ibid.

13. Timothy C. Hain, "Otosclerosis," http://www.dizziness-and balance .com/disorders/hearing/otoscler.html, accessed February 18, 2015.

14. Stevens and Hemingway, "Beethoven's Deafness," 436.

15. A. C. F. Hui and S. M. Wong, "Deafness and Liver Disease in a 57-Year-Old Man: A Medical History of Beethoven," *Hong Kong Medical Journal* 6/4 (December 2000): 435; Sebahattin Cureoglu, Muzeyyen Yildirim Baylan, and Michael M. Paparella, "Cochlear Otosclerosis," *Current Opinion in Otolaryngology & Head and Neck Surgery* 18/5 (October 2010): 357–62.

16. Hui and Wong, "Deafness and Liver Disease," 435. The diagnosis of otosclerosis is described as likely, but not conclusive, in Hans Bankl and Hans Jesserer's documentary study *Die Krankheiten Ludwig van Beethovens* (Vienna: Wilhelm Maudrich, 1987), 124. However, Maurice Scorsby, in "Beethoven's Deafness," *Journal of Laryngology and Otology* 45 (1930): 529–44, claimed that medical knowledge at the time of Beethoven's deafness was sufficient that stapes fixation would have been noted in the autopsy if it had been present, as would other physical traces produced by otosclerosis.

17. In personal correspondence on May 6, 2016, audiologist Marshall Chasin argued against this diagnosis: "Cochlear otosclerosis is extremely rare and I may have seen this once in my 35 year career. Much more likely is that Beethoven may have had two unrelated sources of his loss—otosclerosis (middle ear) and perhaps some lead toxicity leading to a sensory neural component to his hearing."

18. In an appendix to *Beethoven the Creator* (New York: Harper and Brothers, 1929), 265–90, Rolland dismissed all the customary explanations as inadequate to explain the extent of Beethoven's deafness, then cited his correspondence with a French doctor named Marage in support of the comparison with yoga. The reference to Beethoven's "furious concentration" is on p. 278. See also Marage (no first name given), "Causes et conséquences de la surdité de Beethoven," transmitted by d'Arsonvale, *Comptes rendus des séances hebdomadaires de l'Académie des Sciences* 189 (1929): 1036–38.

Solomon, in chapter 6 of his *Beethoven Essays* (Cambridge, MA: Harvard University Press, 1988), 93–98, states that "Beethoven's deafness, whether or not it was 'willed' or generated through some obscure psychosomatic mechanism, served to protect his creativity from the assaults and seductions of the external world and from the memories of a submissive past at a moment when he was about to embark upon what he termed his 'new path,' a path that would lead him to transform the parameters and procedures of the Viennese Classic tradition and to establish new boundaries and norms for the future development of music" (95). Both writers note that withdrawal into a private world was characteristic of Beethoven even during his childhood, and suggest that his deafness has to be understood in connection to this withdrawal and perhaps as a manifestation of it.

19. For a strong argument that Beethoven did have syphilis and that it was the root cause of his deafness, see McCabe, "Beethoven's Deafness." However, this argument was based largely on the idea that he used a salve containing mercury, which has now been proved false. See Michael H. Stevens, Teemarie Jacobsen, and Alicia Kay Crofts, "Lead and the Deafness of Ludwig van Beethoven," *Laryngoscope* 123 (2013): 2855. Paul C. Squires, in "The Problem of Beethoven's Deafness," *Journal of Abnormal and Social Psychology* 32 (1937): 11–62, also argued for syphilis, and for a cover-up by Beethoven's friends and admirers. Squires also provided one of the most extensive surveys available of earlier literature on the cause of Beethoven's deafness.

20. Numerous contemporary accounts of Beethoven's use of alcohol are provided in Bankl and Jesserer, *Die Krankheiten Ludwig van Beethovens*, 75–78.

21. The latter hypothesis is advocated strongly as the cause of Beethoven's deafness in Stevens, Jacobsen, and Crofts, "Lead and the Deafness of Ludwig van Beethoven:" 2854–58. The idea that Beethoven's death was caused by lead poisoning is challenged in Josef Eisinger, "Was Beethoven Lead-Poisoned?," *Beethoven Journal* 23/1 (Summer 2008): 15–17.

22. Hui and Wong, "Deafness and Liver Disease," 436.

23. Collin S. Karmody and Edgar S. Bachor, "The Deafness of Ludwig van

Beethoven: An Immunopathy," *Otology and Neurotology* 26/4 (July 2005): 809–14.

24. A provisional diagnosis of otosclerosis would be supported by the gradual progress of Beethoven's deafness, but here too there are inconsistencies. For one thing, otosclerosis rarely leads to deafness as profound as that in which Beethoven apparently spent the final years of his life. This has caused speculation that he also suffered from Paget's disease, a pathological malformation of the skull, or at least from labyrinthisis chronica ossificans, a rare form of the disease characterized by "diffuse infiltration of the inner ear with otosclerotic bone." See Nehemiah Asherson, "The Deafness of Beethoven and the Saga of the Stapes," *Transactions of the Hunterian Society* 24 (1965–66): 22.

25. Wegeler/Ries, 86.

26. This story is attributed to Ries by Ludwig Rellstab, as quoted in Peter J. Davies, *Beethoven in Person: His Deafness, Illnesses, and Death* (Westport, CT: Greenwood, 2001), 47–48. The full text is given in H. C. Robbins Landon, *Beethoven: A Documentary Study* (London: Thames and Hudson, 1970), 286–87, along with a suggested date of 1804.

27. Wayne Senner, Robin Wallace, and William Meredith, eds., Robin Wallace, trans., *The Critical Reception of Beethoven's Compositions by His German Contemporaries* (Lincoln: University of Nebraska Press, 2001), 2:49. This incident and the subsequent communication to Breitkopf und Härtel are also cited in Ealy, "Of Ear Trumpets," 265. Ealy traces the progress of Beethoven's deafness by citing contemporary sources, and I have drawn on his narrative at several points in this chapter.

28. Brandenburg, *Briefwechsel Gesamtausgabe*, 2:45 (no. 359). My translation. See also Ealy, "Of Ear Trumpets," 265.

29. Ibid., 2:53 (no. 370).

30. The manuscript clearly reads "Violini con sordino," which may be assumed to apply to the viola part as well, but many editions omit this, giving the impression that Beethoven wanted only the cellos to play with mutes, as specified in the letter. This is not the case. The first Breitkopf und Härtel edition does not incorporate Beethoven's change and doesn't show the sordino marking either in any of the parts. This probably explains why it was later incorporated into the cello parts alone.

31. Brandenburg, *Briefwechsel Gesamtausgabe*, 2:118 (no. 439). My translation.

32. Cf. Thayer-Forbes, 473–74. I have altered the English translation, which originally read "Cotton in my ears at the pianoforte frees my hearing from the unpleasant buzzing." This episode is also cited in Ealy, "Of Ear Trumpets," 266, although the dating of the first pages of the Petter sketchbook to as early

as 1809 is no longer accepted; see Douglas Johnson, Alan Tyson, and Robert Winter, *The Beethoven Sketchbooks: History, Reconstruction, Inventory* (Berkeley: University of California Press, 1985), 207–29.

33. Wegeler/Ries, 86.

34. Andreas Ignaz Wawruch, "Medical Review on the Final Stage of L. van Beethoven's Life," trans. Michael Lorenz, *Beethoven Journal* 22/2 (Winter 2007): 88. See also Ealy, "Of Ear Trumpets," 266.

35. Hui and Wong, "Deafness and Liver Disease," 434. One other explanation has been advanced that should be carefully considered, since it would effectively challenge the prevailing view that Beethoven's deafness was caused by otosclerosis. Citing Politzer (see n. 7 above), Peter J. Davies has noted that "deafness is a well recognized complication of meningitis, tending to have its onset after the return of consciousness or during convalescence.... After a rapid onset and progression, there was sometimes a considerable improvement after convalescence, only to be followed months or years later by a progressive severe deafness." See Peter J. Davies, "The Cause of Beethoven's Deafness," in *Aflame with Music: 100 Years of Music at the University of Melbourne*, ed. Brenton Broadstock et al. (Parkville, Victoria: Centre for Studies in Australian Music, 1996), 147. Davies suggested that a diagnosis of meningo-neuro-labyrinthisis is consistent with all of Beethoven's observed symptoms and with the autopsy results (ibid., 147–48). Davies reiterates this conclusion in his book *Beethoven in Person: His Deafness, Illness, and Death* (see n. 26), which also contains an extensive listing of previously suggested diagnoses dating back to Beethoven's own lifetime. If this originated in his unidentified illness of 1796, it would also explain Ries's observation that his hearing improved for a time before growing worse.

36. E.g., the comments by Dr. Karl von Bursy and Fanny Gannatasio cited in Ealy, "Of Ear Trumpets," 267–68.

37. Ryan J. Huxtable, in "The Deafness of Beethoven: A Paradigm of Hearing Problems," *Proceedings of the Western Pharmacology Society* 43 (2000): 1, notes that

> the deaf can appear to comprehend better at one time than another, due to differences in background noise, importance of what is being said, and other factors, leading the uninformed to conclude that the deaf have some control over what they hear. However, hearing is a psychosocial state, and not merely a physical sense. One can hear yet not understand. Or worse, one can hear and misunderstand. Even for those with normal hearing, a high percentage of phonemes are missed, and are filled in mentally. Thus, it is harder to understand a foreign tongue because the ability to supply the missing

phonemes is less developed. For a person whose hearing is impaired, if guesses as to sense are wrong in light social conversation, these are not particularly important. If the subject of conversation is significant, mishearing becomes important. In such a conversation, the deaf person becomes more uncertain as to the accuracy of the aural perceptions. Thus, comprehension is determined by the importance of what is being said.

38. Brandenburg, *Briefwechsel Gesamtausgabe*, 1:85 (no. 67). My translation.

39. Ibid.

40. Ibid., 124n2. The latter's name was consistently left out, apparently due to confusion about which of his given names he wished to be addressed by.

41. Brandenburg, *Briefwechsel Gesamtausgabe*, 1:121 (no. 105). My translation.

42. Wegeler/Ries, 5.

43. Ibid., 149.

44. The astute Alan Tyson called attention to this paradox in a 1969 article in *Musical Times*, in which he also pointed out that the dramatic subjects Beethoven chose at this time—Christ in Gethsemane, Florestan in a basement dungeon—present powerful images of human solitude and isolation. See Alan Tyson, "Beethoven's Heroic Phase," *Musical Times* 110 (February 1969): 139–41. On the close correspondences between *Christus am Oelberge* and the Heiligenstadt Testament, see Theodore Albrecht, "The Fortnight Fallacy: A Revised Chronology for Beethoven's *Christ on the Mount of Olives*, Op. 85, and Wielhorsky Sketchbook," *Journal of Musicological Research* 11 (1991): 1–22; Barry Cooper, "Beethoven's Oratorio and the Heiligenstadt Testament," *Beethoven Journal* 10/1 (Spring 1995): 19–24; and Owen Jander, "The Rhetorical Structure of Beethoven's Heiligenstadt Testament," *Beethoven Journal* 22/1 (Summer 2007): 6–16.

45. This is based on the account of Louis Spohr, who first encountered Beethoven in late 1812. See Thayer/Forbes, 547, and Ealy, "Of Ear Trumpets," 266.

46. Thayer-Forbes, 577; Ealy, "Of Ear Trumpets," 270.

47. Barry Cooper, ed., *The Beethoven Compendium: A Guide to Beethoven's Life and Music* (London: Thames and Hudson, 1991), 24.

48. For an important perspective on these "fallow" years and their creative significance, see Lewis Lockwood, "The Three Years 1813–1817: A 'Fallow' Period in Beethoven's Career?," in *Beiträge zu Biographie und Schaffensprozess bei Beethoven, Rainer Cadenbach zum Gedenken*, ed. Jürgen May (Bonn: Verlag Beethoven-Haus, 2011), 89–99.

49. Alice Miller, *The Drama of the Gifted Child*, translated from the German by Ruth Ward (New York: Basic Books, 1990), 5–6.

50. Ealy, "Of Ear Trumpets," 273.

51. The "Nachrichten" section of *Allgemeine musikalische Zeitung* 18/8 (February 21, 1816) states in column 121 that "this great artist is much to be pitied, as he is losing more and more of his hearing, which tragic circumstance makes him nearly incapable of directing the performance of his works on his own." Shortly after Beethoven's death, strong denunciations of his late music appeared in the *Allgemeine musikalische Zeitung* and in the rival periodical *Caecilia*; the authors of both took it for granted that what they saw as the poor quality of the music could be ascribed to his deafness. See Robin Wallace, *Beethoven's Critics: Aesthetic Dilemmas and Resolutions during the Composer's Lifetime* (Cambridge: Cambridge University Press, 1986), 41–42, 66–69.

52. See the descriptions of Beethoven's improvising in 1823 by Friedrich Wieck and in 1824 by Johann Andreas Stumpff, in Klaus Martin Kopitz and Rainer Cadenbach, eds., *Beethoven aus der Sicht seiner Zeitgenossen in Tagebüchern, Briefen, Gedichten und Erinnerungen* (Munich: G. Henle, 2009), 2:1094 and 2:975, respectively. These will be discussed further in chapter 5. See also Ealy, "Of Ear Trumpets," 272.

53. Ealy, "Of Ear Trumpets," 268–70.

54. Samuel Heinrich Spiker, who visited Beethoven in 1826, recounts seeing several sketchbooks on the desk next to the Graf piano that Beethoven was using at the time. See Kopitz and Cadenbach, *Beethoven aus der Sicht seiner Zeitgenossen*, 2:927. See also Ealy, "Of Ear Trumpets," 272.

55. The resonator and Beethoven's use of it are described in Ealy, "Of Ear Trumpets, 271–73, although Ealy gets many details wrong, including missing the fact that the original resonator was built for the Broadwood, not the Graf. For further details on this important device, see chapter 5.

56. Friedrich August Kanne, "Performance of Mr. Ludwig van Beethoven," *Allgemeine musikalische Zeitung mit besonderer Rücksicht auf den österreichischen Kaiserstaat* 8 (June 5, 9, and 16, 1824), in *The Critical Reception of Beethoven's Compositions by His German Contemporaries, Op. 125*, ed. and trans. Robin Wallace (Boston: Center for Beethoven Studies, Boston University, 2017), 9, http://www.bu.edu/beethovencenter/files/2017/06/robinwallace-publication.pdf.

57. Quoted in Thayer-Forbes, 940–41.

58. Similar passages can arguably be found in m. 5 of the introduction to this movement, in mm. 85–87 of the first movement of the sonata in A major, op. 101, and in mm. 165–72 of the second movement of the *Hammerklavier* sonata, op. 106, although in the latter two cases the dynamic peak is marked *fortissimo*.

59. Franz Dotter and Ingeborg Okorn, "Austria's Hidden Conflict: Hearing Culture versus Deaf Culture," in *Many Ways to Be Deaf: International Variation*

in Deaf Communities, ed. Leila Frances Monaghan et al. (Washington, DC: Gallaudet University Press, 2003), 49–50.

CHAPTER TWO

1. Oliver Sacks, *Migraine: Understanding a Common Disorder,* rev. ed. (Berkeley: University of California Press, 1985), 108.

2. Ibid.

3. For details on the anatomy of this part of the ear, see Thierry Mom et al., "Cochlear Blood Supply: An Update on Anatomy and Function," *Fr ORL* 2005: 81–88, http://citeseerx.ist.psu.edu/viewdoc/download?doi=10.1.1.472.3787& rep=rep1&type=pdf, accessed October 21, 2017.

CHAPTER THREE

1. Robert Gjerdingen, *Music in the Galant Style* (Oxford: Oxford University Press, 2007), 333.

2. Gjerdingen's *Music in the Galant Style* (ibid.) provides an extensive description of this style and its defining characteristics. Gjerdingen argues that the historiography of eighteenth-century music would be better served by de-emphasizing the traditional labels *baroque* and *classical* and focusing on Italy rather than on Germany.

3. Ibid., 8–10.

4. In an important essay on *Fidelio* that appeared in the *Allgemeine musikalische Zeitung* in 1815, the German philosopher and critic Amadeus Wendt expressed reservations about Beethoven's instrumental music. "Many works of Beethoven, for example, various symphonies and sonatas of his, can only be understood and evaluated as *musical fantasies.* In them, even the attentive listener often completely loses sight of the fundamental idea." Senner, Wallace, and Meredith, *Critical Reception,* 2:199. A critic of the *Harp* Quartet, op. 74, wrote in 1811 that "the minimal melodic coherence, and the humorous wandering back and forth from one idea to another, gives it more the appearance of a free fantasy than of an orderly whole." ("Recension: Quatour pour 2 Violons, Viola et Violencelle comp.—par L. v. Beethoven. Oeuv. 74. A Leipsic, chet Breitkopf et Härtel [Preis 1 Thlr. 8 Gr.])," *Allgemeine musikalische Zeitung* 13 [May 1811]: 349–51.) By contrast, a review of the Fantasy in G Minor for Piano, op. 77, makes it clear that the standards applied to other types of composition did not apply to a work of this type: "As broken off and disjointed as its individual movements appear to be at first glance, they nevertheless stand in the most

beautiful harmonic connectedness, and form a magnificent whole, which one would not hesitate to put forward as the model for the fantasy, if it did not contradict the character and the essence of this type of music to wish to prescribe a specific form for it." ("Rezensionen neuer Musikalien: Fantaisie pour le Pianoforte composée et dediée—par L. v. Beethoven Oeuv. 77 à Vienne chez Jean Cappi," *Wiener allgemeine musikalische Zeitung* 1 [March 27, 1813]: 197–99). The difference between a fantasy (improvisation) and a work in a more established genre is clarified in a review of op. 80, the Fantasy for Piano, Choir, and Orchestra: "The fantasy is the artist's monologue, in which he purely expresses his individual, personal experience, whereas he can only relate to given forms—to the oratorio, to the opera, and so forth—in dialogue. . . . If, constrained by established forms to speak only in accordance with them, it becomes more or less necessary for him to alloy himself with foreign matter, and to take up foreign material into his creation, then in free fantasy, on the contrary, all fetters are broken, and the artist's genius is placed back in its proper domain, older than the forms, as creator and lord in the kingdom of sounds." ("Recension: Phantasie für das Pianoforte, mit Begleitung des ganzen Orchesters und Chor, in Musik gesetzt——von Louis van Beethoven. 80stes Werk [Eigenthum der Verleger.] Leipzig, bey Breitkopf und Härtel [Preis 2 Thlr. 12 Gr.]," *Allgemeine musikalische Zeitung* 13 [May 1812]: 307–11.) The translations given here are my own.

5. "Schreiben Mozarts an den Baron von . . . ," *Allgemeine musikalische Zeitung* 17 (August 23, 1815): 563–64. My translation.

6. (New York: Dover, 1967). The resemblances between the two passages, and the spurious nature of both, are discussed in detail in Maynard Solomon, "On Beethoven's Creative Process: A Two-Part Invention," *Music and Letters* 61 (1980): 272–83.

7. The term *pianoforte*, meaning an instrument that can play both soft and loud, has been in use since the 18th century and is sometimes used to designate historical instruments, as is the term *fortepiano*, also widely used at that time. For the sake of clarity I use *piano*, the common modern usage, exclusively in the text.

8. Tilman Skowroneck, "The Keyboard Instruments of the Young Beethoven," in *Beethoven and His World*, ed. Scott Burnham and Michael P. Steinberg (Princeton: Princeton University Press, 2000), 157–58.

9. Ibid., 162–72. Skowroneck provides a great deal of valuable information in these pages about Beethoven's personal preferences, descriptions of his playing, and his correspondence with piano manufacturers, with whom he did not always see eye to eye. See also Skowroneck's *Beethoven the Pianist* (Cambridge:

Cambridge University Press, 2010), where he affirms on p. 74 that "Beethoven and [Viennese piano manufacturer Andreas] Streicher agreed that it was the player's responsibility to learn to make the piano 'sing' and to avoid letting it sound like a 'tinkling harp.'"

10. Beethoven used this phrase in a letter to the piano manufacturer Andreas Streicher quoted in ibid., 171. See chapter 5 here for further specifics.

11. Friedrich Schneider (1786–1853), who played the premiere of the *Emperor* Concerto in 1811, was said by Beethoven's biographer Ludwig Nohl to have visited Beethoven in 1819. Nohl reported that "the master even 'improvised' [*phantasirt*] at his invitation: it was the best thing he had ever heard, much better than all of his works. Even in recounting this Schneider became very exhilarated. And Beethoven himself was so touched by the playing that on standing up he knocked over a table with an expensive tea set." Kopitz and Cadenbach, *Beethoven aus der Sicht seiner Zeitgenossen*, 2:835, my translation. There is a brief report in *Allgemeine musikalische Zeitung* 24 (1822): 310, under the heading "Miscellen," stating that Beethoven had recently improvised several times in a masterly way in a social setting to the joy of all present, "and demonstrated that he still understands how to handle his instrument with vigor, joy, and love." Friedrich Wieck heard Beethoven improvise in 1823 and was highly impressed (Kopitz and Cadenbach, *Beethoven aus der Sicht seiner Zeitgenossen*, 2:1094), as was Johann Stumpff the following year. Stumpff managed to suggest simultaneously that Beethoven improvised brilliantly and that he tormented his mangled Broadwood piano in the process (ibid., 2:975). Wieck's report of his visit also appears in O. G. Sonneck, ed., *Beethoven: Impressions by His Contemporaries* (New York: Dover, 1967), 207–9, where it is incorrectly dated 1824 or 1826, leading Ealy, in "Of Ear Trumpets," to give 1826 as the date.

12. Skowroneck, "Keyboard Instruments of the Young Beethoven," 152. Skowroneck argues persuasively against the views of several earlier writers who have seen dissatisfaction with the instruments at his disposal as a determining feature of Beethoven's approach to the piano.

13. Joseph Kerman, "Beethoven's Early Sketches," *Musical Quarterly* 56 (1970): 538.

14. William S. Newman, *Beethoven on Beethoven: Playing His Piano Music His Way* (New York: W. W. Norton, 1988), 34–35.

15. Solomon, "On Beethoven's Creative Process," 273.

16. Ibid., 273–74.

17. I am grateful to Eleanor Smith of the Orpheus Institute for the suggestion that Beethoven could have gone through a similar process in his sketches.

18. Kerman, "Beethoven's Early Sketchesm" 522–23.

19. Samuel Heinrich Spiker, who visited Beethoven that year, described Beethoven's pocket sketchbooks and went on to say that "various large books of this kind lay on the desk next to his pianoforte, in which lengthy fragments of music were written in ink." Kopitz and Cadenbach, *Beethoven aus der Sicht seiner Zeitgenossen*, 2:927, my translation. Clearly Beethoven was still working at the piano. See also Ealy, "Of Ear Trumpets," 273.

20. Ernst Woldemar, "Aufforderung an die Redaktion der Cäcilia," *Caecilia* 8 (1828): 36–40, and an anonymous article titled "Einige Worte zu den vielen über Beethovens letzte Werke," *Allgemeine musikalische Zeitung* 31 (April 29, 1829): 269–73.

21. Woldemar, "Aufforderung:" 37, 39. My translation.

22. See K. M. Knittel, "Wagner, Deafness, and the Reception of Beethoven's Late Style," *Journal of the American Musicological Society* 51 (1998): 51–54.

23. Ibid., 49–82. Maynard Solomon, in 1990, staked out a similar position to that of Wagner, claiming that "Beethoven's deafness . . . served to protect his creativity from the assaults and seductions of the external world and from the memories of a submissive past at a moment when he was about to embark upon what he termed his 'new path,' a path that would lead him to transform the parameters and procedures of the Viennese Classic tradition and to establish new boundaries and norms for the future development of music." "On Beethoven's Deafness," in *Beethoven Essays* (Cambridge: Harvard University Press, 1988), 95. More recently Megan Ross, in "Beethoven's Late Quartets and Wagner's 1870 'Beethoven' Essay Revisited," a paper delivered at the Seventh New Beethoven Research Conference, Rochester, NY, 2017, pointed out that Beethoven's deafness began to be interpreted as a creative advantage in reviews of his late music as early as 1825.

24. Nicholas Cook, *Music: A Very Short Introduction* (Oxford: Oxford University Press, 1998), 22–23.

25. See, for example, Friedrich August Kanne, "Performance of Mr. Ludwig van Beethoven," *Allgemeine musikalische Zeitung mit besonderer Rücksicht auf den österreichischen Kaiserstaat* 8 (1824): 149–51, 157–60, 173–74, in *The Critical Reception of Beethoven's Compositions by His German Contemporaries, op. 125*, ed. and trans. Robin Wallace (Boston: Center for Beethoven Studies, Boston University, 2017), 8-20, http://www.bu.edu/beethovencenter/files/2017/06/robinwallace-publication.pdf., the review by Ignaz Xaver Seyfried of the *Missa Solemnis*, the Ninth Symphony, and the String Quartet op. 131 in *Caecilia* 9 (1828): 217–43, the reviews of the *Missa Solemnis* by Georg Christian Grossheim and Joseph Fröhlich in *Caecilia* 9 (1828): 22–45, the reviews of the

Ninth Symphony by the same two writers in *Caecilia* 9 (1828): 231–61, translated in Wallace, *Critical Reception of Beethoven's Compositions*, 58-27, and the commentary on op. 131 by Friedrich Rochlitz in *Allgemeine musikalische Zeitung* 30 (1828): 485–95, 501–9.

26. Senner, Wallace, and Meredith, *Critical Reception*, v2:2, 20.

27. Ibid., 15.

28. For example, even Amadeus Wendt (see n. 4, above) saw in much of Beethoven's music "a bold flight of fantasy that in itself carries the foundation of its downfall and a straining of the feeling, which does not admit of a long duration and with closer contact with reality must necessarily become languor." Senner, Wallace, and Meredith, *Critical Reception*, 2:201. Waldemar Schweisheimer, in *Beethovens Leiden: Ihr Einfluss auf sein Leben und Schaffen* (Munich: Georg Müller, 1922), esp. 111–12, argued that that the perceived failings in Beethoven's later music that have been blamed on his deafness—ungracious vocal writing, loud instrumentation, and awkward writing for instruments—were already largely present in his earlier music, when Beethoven could have corrected them but chose not to do so.

29. Joseph Fröhlich, "First Review," *Caecilia* 8 (1828), in *Critical Reception of Beethoven's Compositions*, ed. and trans. Wallace.

CHAPTER FOUR

1. Thayer-Forbes, 730. The original reference is in Anton Schindler, "Zur Beantwortung der Fragen über Beethoven's Taubheit, in Nr. 54 dieses Blattes," *Niederrheinische Musik-Zeitung für Kunstfreunde und Künstler* 2 (1854): 224. Schindler's contribution, which begins on the previous page, provides a wealth of information, all of which is subject to the usual reservations about the author's trustworthiness.

2. Post to ClarionCI@yahoogroups.com, February 22, 2004.

3. That Beethoven had the same problem is documented in Grita Herre, ed., *Beethoven im Gespräch: Ein Konversationsheft vom 9. September 1825* (Bonn: Verlag Beethoven-Haus, 2002), 63 (German original) and 95 (English translation).

4. One of the best overviews of the early history and development of the cochlear implant can be found in Stuart Blume, *The Artificial Ear: Cochlear Implants and the Culture of Deafness* (New Brunswick, NJ: Rutgers University Press, 2010), 30–57. Blume's book as a whole problematizes the apparent success of cochlear implantation, particularly in children, by situating it within the context of the Deaf community's lack of influence on the ways in which that success is understood.

5. A detailed description of implantation surgery and its aftermath can be found in Michael Chorost's book *Rebuilt: My Journey Back to the Hearing World* (Boston: Houghton-Mifflin, 2005; the book has also been marketed with the subtitle *How Becoming Part Computer Made Me More Human*). Chorost writes from the perspective of someone who had been hard of hearing since birth but suddenly—though not as suddenly as Barbara—lost what was left of his hearing as an adult. His implant, like Barbara's, was manufactured by the firm Advanced Bionics, one of only a handful of companies that make them. In reading his account of the aftermath of implantation, I was struck by the strong parallels to Barbara's experience, some of which those familiar with Chorost's book may recognize in the pages that follow.

6. Post to ClarionCI@yahoogroups.com, June 23, 2004.

7. Maynard Solomon, "Beethoven's Tagebuch," in *Beethoven Essays*, 260.

8. Timbre—the quality of a sound—is what distinguishes one sound from another when other factors like pitch and volume are discounted. The ability to pick out certain timbres allowed Barbara to know that she was hearing a piano or a wind instrument even if she was unable to tell what that instrument was playing.

9. https://www.advancedbionics.com/content/advancedbionics/com/en/home/products/sound-processing/hires-fidelity-120.html, accessed November 4, 2017. The process described here under "Simultaneous Stimulation is the Secret" is the same one used for the Harmony processor.

10. Michael Chorost (see fn. 5 in this chapter) reports on an experiment with what must have been an early version of this software in "My Bionic Quest for Boléro," *Wired*, November 1, 2005, http://www.wired.com/2005/11/bolero/, accessed October 26, 2017. Like Barbara, he was both pleased and disappointed with the results.

11. Lockwood and Gosman, *Beethoven's "Eroica" Sketchbook*, 1:32–35.

12. Ibid., 1:34.

13. Post to ClarionCI@yahoogroups.com, April 27, 2006.

CHAPTER FIVE

1. See Johnson, Tyson, and Winter, *Beethoven Sketchbooks*.

2. See, for example, Joseph Kerman, ed., *Ludwig van Beethoven. Autograph Miscellany from circa 1786 to 1799: British Museum Additional Manuscript no. 29801, ff. 39–162 (The Kafka Sketchbook)* (London: British Museum, 1970); William Kinderman, ed., *Artaria 195: Beethoven's Sketchbook for the "Missa*

Solemnis" and the Piano Sonata in E Major, Opus 109, 3 vols. (Urbana: University of Illinois Press, 2003); and Lewis Lockwood and Alan Gosman, eds., *Beethoven's "Eroica" Sketchbook: A Critical Edition,* 2 vols. (Urbana: University of Illinois Press, 2013).

3. The largest single collection of sketches and manuscripts can be found at the website of the Beethoven-Haus in Bonn: http://www.beethoven-haus -bonn.de/sixcms/detail.php?id=1509&template=einstieg_digitales_archiv _en&_mid=Sketches%20by%20%20Beethoven. For examples of print publications of Beethoven's manuscripts, see Alan Tyson, ed., *Beethoven: String Quartet Opus 59 No. 1 (First "Razumovsky" Quartet, in F major)* (London: Scolar Press, 1980); and Lewis Lockwood, *Beethoven: Studies in the Creative Process* (Cambridge, MA: Harvard University Press, 1992), which contains a facsimile of the entire first movement of the cello sonata, op. 69, in manuscript.

A list of Beethoven manuscripts that are available online can be found at the website of the Center for Beethoven Research at Boston University: http://www.bu.edu/beethovencenter/beethoven-autographs-online/.

4. Haydn's working method is discussed in great detail, and his use of these terms clarified, in Hollace Ann Schafer, "'A Wisely Ordered *Phantasie*': Joseph Haydn's Creative Process from the Sketches and Drafts for Instrumental Music" (PhD diss., Brandeis University, 1987).

5. Alan Gosman, "Page Folds in Landsberg 6," in *Beethoven's "Eroica" Sketchbook,* transcr. and ed. Lewis Lockwood and Alan Gosman (Urbana: University of Illinois Press, 2013), 1:14–19.

6. Brandenburg, *Briefwechsel Gesamuausgabe,* 3:20 (no. 707). My translation.

7. Kopitz and Cadenbach, *Beethoven aus der Sicht seiner Zeitgenossen,* 1:18. "Zwei bis drei Flügel, alle ohne Beine auf der Erde liegend . . ."

8. Brian F. McCabe, in "Beethoven's Deafness," 201–2, points out that the only source for this story is "an obscure French physician named J. A. A. Rattel, who could not have observed it first-hand because he was not a contemporary of Beethoven's. The master may have experimented with it briefly but it could not have been his practice, since it totally escapes mention by his multitude of biographers and correspondents." See also Ealy, "Of Ear Trumpets," 271. A claim by Raoul Blondel that Beethoven used a wooden cylinder that he touched to his ear at one end and to the instrument at the other, and which was the ancestor of the modern stethoscope, is likewise unsubstantiated. See Raoul Blondel, "La surdité de Beethoven," *Le ménestrel* 90 (1928): 174.

9. The rhetorical aspects of playing Haydn's music on eighteenth-century

instruments are discussed extensively by Tom Beghin, most recently in *The Virtual Haydn: Paradox of a Twenty-First-Century Keyboardist* (Chicago: University of Chicago Press, 2015).

10. For a detailed statistical study of some of the important features of early pianos, see Kenneth Mobbs, "A Performer's Comparative Study of Touchweight, Key-Dip, Keyboard Design and Repetition in Early Grand Pianos, c. 1770 to 1850," *Galpin Society Journal* 54 (May 2001): 16–54.

11. A good resource on the early history of the piano is Edwin M. Good, *Giraffes, Black Dragons, and Other Pianos: A Technological History from Cristofori to the Modern Concert Grand,* 2nd ed. (Stanford, CA: Stanford University Press, 2001).

12. For a detailed description of the Viennese "Prellmechanik," the English "Stoßmechanik," and the differences between them, see Tom Beghin, "Three Builders, Two Pianos, One Pianist: The Told and Untold Story of Ignaz Moscheles's Concert on 15 December 1823," *19th-Century Music* 24 (2000): 137–38.

13. Brandenburg, *Briefwechsel Gesamuausgabe*, 1, 3:33 (no. 23). My translation.

14. Skowroneck, "Keyboard Instruments of the Young Beethoven," 172–76.

15. Tilman Skowroneck, "Beethoven's Erard Piano: Its Influence on His Compositions and on Viennese Fortepiano Building," *Early Music* 30 (2002): 523. See also Tia DeNora, *Beethoven and the Construction of Genius: Musical Politics in Vienna, 1792–1803* (Berkeley: University of California Press, 1995), 174–79.

16. Good, *Giraffes, Black Dragons, and Other Pianos,* 93.

17. A glissando is an effect in which one of the pianist's fingers slides over a series of keys, causing them to sound quickly in succession. This effect is still easy to produce on a modern piano, but in the passage in question Beethoven asks the pianist to play two slides an octave apart with the same hand; modern pianos have made this considerably more difficult to do.

18. See, for example, Tilman Skowroneck, "A Brit in Vienna: Beethoven's Broadwood Piano," *Keyboard Perspectives* 5 (2012): 42. In his book *Beethoven the Pianist* (Cambridge: Cambridge University Press, 2010), Skowroneck argues persuasively against the commonly held view that Beethoven had always sought to exceed the limits of the instruments he had available. As he points out, credible evidence about broken strings and instrument abuse arises only after increasing deafness began to curtail his performing career.

19. Skowroneck, *Beethoven the Pianist,* 86.

20. Good, *Giraffes, Black Dragons, and Other Pianos,* 97.

21. Skowroneck, *Beethoven the Pianist,* 99.

22. Ibid., 88–103. Skowroneck relates a large amount of specific information about the nature of the changes that were made, which tends to suggest that they were done in a spirit of increasing desperation.

23. Ibid., 103–15. Further support for the close integration of the *Waldstein* with the sound and action of the Erard is provided in Maria Rose, "New Insights into Beethoven's 'Waldstein' Sonata Op. 53: A Showpiece for Paris," paper delivered at the annual meeting of the American Musicological Society, Pittsburgh, 2013.

24. Cf. Skowroneck, *Beethoven the Pianist*, 113.

25. This effect and other aspects of the instrument's sonority can be observed on Alexei Lubimov's recording of the *Waldstein* on a reconstructed 1802 Erard (Alpha 194, released by Alpha Productions, Paris, in 2012).

26. Thanks to Tom Beghin for confirming the stunning effect of this music, and also of passages from the first movement of the *Waldstein*, when played on the Erard with the *una corda* pedal (personal communication, June 24, 2017).

27. Newman, *Beethoven on Beethoven*, 63.

28. This is suggested in Skowroneck, *Beethoven the Pianist*, 99–103. "It is possible, even likely, that the Érard was a good and powerful piano when new, and that Beethoven's initial 'enchantment' was genuine. It is just as likely that the quality deteriorated noticeably and steadily due to the way he began to treat this piano. This decline in quality would in its turn explain his later dismissal of the instrument" (103).

29. "My Heiligenstadt, of Sorts," posted on Facebook January 12, 2013.

30. Personal communication, February 19, 2015.

31. Ibid.

32. Tellingly, the website of the Hyperacusis Network warns that "those who come down with hyperacusis may overprotect their ears because they have a fear of noise (phonophobia). For those who suddenly develop severe hyperacusis, it may be necessary to use ear protection so that the patient's ears have an opportunity to regroup and recover. After a few months however, over protection will only further collapse ones tolerance to sound. The patient is in a Catch 22 and walks a fine line between over protecting and under protecting their ears. Most, over a period of time learn to trust their instincts." Hyperacusis Network, Decreased Sound Tolerance, http://www.hyperacusis.net/what-to-do/, accessed July 26, 2017.

33. For a persuasive argument in support of this view, see Beverly Jerold, "Mälzel's Role in Beethoven's Symphonic Metronome Marks," in *Music Performance Issues: 1600–1900* (Hillsdale, NY: Pendragon, 2016), 165–92.

34. Ibid., 165–66.

35. Thayer-Forbes, 543. For more on Mälzel's early career see Rita Steblin, "Mälzel's Early Career to 1813: New Archival Research in Regensburg and Vienna," in *Colloquium Collegarum: Festschrift für David Hiley zum 65. Geburtstag*, ed. Wolfgang Horn and Fabian Weber (Tutzing: Hans Schneider, 2013), 161–210.

36. As we will see, Beethoven also used the terms *gehör Maschine* (hearing machine), *Ohrenmaschine* (ear machine), and *Sprachrohr* (speaking tube). An anonymous writer in 1854 who claimed to have known Beethoven used the term *Ohrentrichter* (ear funnel). See "Ueber Beethoven's Taubheit," *Niederrheinische Musik-Zeitung für Kunstfreunde und Künstler* 2 (1854): 213.

37. Mara Mills, "When Mobile Communication Technologies Were New," *Endeavour* 33/4 (2009): 142.

38. Elisabeth Bennion, *Antique Hearing Devices* (London: Vernier, 1994), 6–7.

39. Mary Lou Koelkebeck, Colleen Detjen, and Donald R. Calvert, *Historic Devices for Hearing: The CID-Goldstein Collection* (Saint Louis, MO: Central Institute for the Deaf, 1984), 10.

40. Four of these devices, including the two with resonators, are on display at the Beethoven-Haus in Bonn. The fifth is in the possession of the Gesellschaft der Musikfreunde in Vienna.

41. Mills, "When Mobile Communication Technologies Were New," 142.

42. Ibid., 143.

43. Bennion, *Antique Hearing Devices*, 16; Mills, "When Mobile Communication Technologies Were New," 142.

44. Bennion, *Antique Hearing Devices*, 26–27.

45. Mills, "When Mobile Communication Technologies Were New," 142.

46. Thayer-Forbes, 691.

47. Brandenburg, *Briefwechsel Gesamuausgabe*, 3:5 (no. 691). My translation.

48. Ealy, "Of Ear Trumpets," 266–67, gives further details of the quarrel between Beethoven and Mälzel, which also involved two orchestral concerts given by Mälzel without Beethoven's approval. As Ealy points out, Schindler's claim that Beethoven only found one of Mälzel's ear trumpets serviceable also needs to be evaluated in this context. See Anton Schindler, *Biographie von Ludwig van Beethoven* (Münster: Aschendorff, 1840), 91. "Nach und nach wurden auch vier Gehörmaschinen fertig, von denen Beethoven aber nur eine brauchbar fand, und sich ihrer durch längere Zeit, besonders bei seinen Zusammenkünften mit dem Erzherzog Rudolph und Anderen, wo die schriftliche Conversation die Unerhaltung verzögerte, bedient hat."

49. See "Recensionen," *Wellington's Sieg, oder, die Schlacht bey Vittoria,*

in Musik gesetzt, und Sr. königl. Hoheit, dem Prinzen Regenten von England—zugeeignet, von Ludwig van Beethoven. 91stes Werk. Vollständige Partitur. (Und die mannigfaltigen Ausgaben, wie sie in der Folge angeführt werden.) Wien, bey S. A. Steiner und Comp., so wie auch in den vorzüglichsten Musikhandlungen Deutschlands, der Schweiz, und Italiens." *Allgemeine musikalische Zeitung* 18 (April 10, 1816): 241–50. This review of the first publication describes Beethoven's written instructions, which were reprinted in both the old and new collected editions of his works.

50. The complete text of Beethoven's *Tagebuch*, as transmitted in a manuscript copy made in 1827 by Anton Gräffer (1784–ca.1849), is given, along with translations and commentary, in Maynard Solomon, "Beethoven's Tagebuch of 1812–1818," in *Beethoven Studies 3*, ed. Alan Tyson, 193–285 (Cambridge: Cambridge University Press, 1982). The passages cited are on pp. 226 and 233. See also Ealy, "Of Ear Trumpets," 267.

51. Brandenburg, *Briefwechsel Gesamuausgabe*, 4:115 (no. 1177). See also Ealy, "Of Ear Trumpets," 268.

52. Gottfried Weber, "Ueber Tonmalerei," *Caecilia* 3, no. 10 (1825): 125–72. Weber's comments originally appeared in the *Jenaischer allgemeine Literaturzeitung* in 1816. We know Beethoven read them when they appeared in *Caecilia* because he responded, "Pitiful scoundrel, my shit is better than [anything] you have ever thought." (See William Kinderman, *Beethoven* [Berkeley: University of California Press, 1995], 180.) We can only speculate about whether he saw them when they first appeared in print almost ten years earlier.

53. Ibid., 167–68.

54. In the conversation books, others would refer to the resonator that was built for his Broadwood piano as a "hearing machine," but the ear trumpets were always *Rohre* (tubes).

55. Köhler and Herre, *Ludwig van Beethovens Konversationshefte*, 1:360.

56. See nn. 79 and 80, below, for a clarification of the details of Kloeber's visit, which has traditionally been described as taking place in 1818.

57. Kopitz and Cadenbach, *Beethoven aus der Sicht seiner Zeitgenossen*, 2:803–4.

58. Graphs showing the results of these tests are reproduced in Koelkebeck et al., *Historic Devices for Hearing*, 27–41. Other types of early hearing aids were also tested, with the results shown elsewhere in the book.

59. Lawrence Yule, "Cupped Hand Amplification," Solent Acoustics, accessed March 29, 2017, https://solentacoustics.wordpress.com/2014/06/17/cupped-hand-amplification/.

60. Newman, *Beethoven on Beethoven*, 45–46.

61. Skowroneck, "Brit in Vienna," 43.

62. Ibid., 44.

63. The one exception is C#7 in the last movement of op. 109, but as Tom Beghin points out in "Beethoven's Broadwood, Stein's Hearing Machine, and a Trilogy of Sonatas," in *Inside the Hearing Machine: Beethoven on His Broadwood, Piano Sonatas Opus 109, 110, and 111* [no editor listed] (N.p.: Evil Penguin Records Classic, 2017), 43–45, Beethoven could have tuned the C7 key a half step sharp to play this note, since there is no C-natural in this octave in the sonata.

64. Tom first suggested this to me during a private conversation in Waco during the fall of 2014; see p. 226.

65. Here, too, I am indebted to Tom Beghin for alerting me to these aspects of the instrument before I had a chance to try it myself.

66. Tom Beghin, "Beethoven's *Hammerklavier* Sonata, Opus 106: Legend, Difficulty, and the Gift of a Broadwood Piano," *Keyboard Perspectives* 7 (2014): 117.

67. Beghin, "Beethoven's Broadwood, Stein's Hearing Machine, and a Trilogy of Sonatas," 46.

68. I am indebted to Tom Beghin for pointing out these acoustical details.

69. The information in this and the succeeding paragraphs is partially based on Skowroneck, "Brit in Vienna," 53–60, titled "Matthäus Andreas Stein and the Hearing Machine, 1820," and on personal correspondence with Tilman Skowroneck. I am also grateful to Theodore Albrecht for sharing portions of his forthcoming edition of the conversation books. Much of the relevant material from the conversation books is reproduced, with a different translation and somewhat different chronology, in *Inside the Hearing Machine*, 82–90.

70. Theodore Albrecht, trans. and ed., *Beethoven's Conversation Books*, 12 vols. (Martlesham, Suffolk, UK: Boydell and Brewer, forthcoming beginning fall 2018), Heft 8, Blatt 33r, 35v.

71. Köhler and Herre, *Ludwig van Beethovens Konversationshefte*, 1:336.

72. Ibid., 1:360–62.

73. Albrecht, *Beethoven's Conversation Books*, Heft 11, Blatt 23r.

74. Ibid., Heft 12, Blatt 25v.

75. Ibid., Heft 12, Blatt 43v.

76. Köhler and Herre, *Ludwig van Beethovens Konversationshefte*, 2:151.

77. Ibid., 2:241.

78. Ibid., 2:244.

79. Kloeber's visit is usually said to have taken place in 1818, but this dating needs to be reconsidered. The editor who printed this story in 1864 identified the place as Mödling, where Beethoven spent several summers, and the year

as 1817. Since Beethoven did not receive the Broadwood until 1818, however, this is clearly incorrect. The hearing machine was not installed until September 1820, so Skowroneck assumes, contrary to conventional wisdom, that the correct year must be 1821 or later, even though Beethoven did not summer in Mödling after 1820. (Skowroneck, "Brit in Vienna," 59). Karl, however, visited Beethoven at Mödling in the late summer of 1820 during a school vacation and remained there until early October (Thayer-Forbes, 764), so it is likely that Kloeber's visit occurred in mid- to late September of that year.

80. *Allgemeine musikalische Zeitung*, n.f. 2, no. 18 (May 4, 1824): 324–25. "Beethoven setzte sich nun, und der Junge musste auf dem Flügel üben, der ein Geschenk aus England war und mit einer grossen Blechkuppel versehen war. Das Instrument stand ungefähr 4–5 Schritten hinter ihn und Beethoven corrigirte dem Jungen, trotz seiner Taubheit, jeden Fehler, liess ihn Einzelnes wiederholen etc."

81. K. M. Knittel, "Pilgrimages to Beethoven: Reminiscences by His Contemporaries," *Music and Letters* 84 (2003): 19–54.

82. Kopitz and Cadenbach, *Beethoven aus der Sicht seiner Zeitgenossen*, 2:1094. It is clear that the "hearing machine" described here was either Stein's original resonator or a later version of it. It was clearly not an ear trumpet, a mistake widely encouraged by O. G. Sonneck's mistranslation of Wieck's account (Sonneck, *Beethoven: Impressions by His Contemporaries*, 207–9), which has in turn been quoted by later writers.

83. Ibid., 2:978n20. "Einem großen Halbwinkel von Resonanz-Holz, welcher an beiden Enden zugemacht war und sich über den Tasten des Klaviers, vom Baß bis zum Diskant erhob, so, daß der Kopf des Spielenden von der Höhe des Halbcirkels eingehüllt war . . ."

84. Ibid., 2:927. "Einer Art von Schallbehälter, unter dem er saß, wenn er spielte, und der dazu dienen sollte, den Schall um ihn her aufzufangen und zu contentriren . . ." See also Ealy, "Of Ear Trumpets," 272. This echoes the description by Gerhard von Breuning, who called it "a sound catcher, placed over the keyboard and the hammers, like a bent sound board built from soft, thin wood, similar to a prompt box: an attempt to direct the instrument's sound waves to the player's ear in more concentrated form." Gerhard von Breuning, *Aus dem Schwarzspanierhause: Erinnerungen an L. van Beethoven aus seiner Jugendzeit*, Neudruck mit Ergänzungen und Erläuterungen von Dr. Alfr. Chr. Kalischer (Berlin: Schuster und Loeffler, 1907), 90. My translation.

85. Wulfrank continued to experiment with the design of the resonator in the months that followed my visit, leading to the version that was used on Tom Beghin's recording, which was intended to optimize the recorded sound

but did not correspond exactly to any of the versions described by Beethoven's contemporaries. Wulfrank also carefully documented the vibrational effects of the instrument that I describe in this chapter. See Thomas Wulfrank, "The Acoustics of Beethoven's Hearing Machine," in *Inside the Hearing Machine*, 58–75.

86. For a detailed discussion of the source material for this sonata, including the probable dates when Beethoven worked on it, see Nicholas Marston, *Beethoven's Piano Sonata in E, Op. 109* (Oxford: Clarendon, 1995), 15–45.

87. Marston, *Beethoven's Piano Sonata in E*, 219 (table 9.1).

88. Ibid., 41.

89. Ibid., 191–92. Note that the label "Var:2" is reserved for a two-measure incipit on the next page.

CHAPTER SIX

1. "Colors," *Radiolab*, season 10, episode 13, http://www.radiolab.org/story/211119-colors/.

2. Marshall Chasin, "Music, Speech and Hearing Devices," in *Making Music with a Hearing Loss: Strategies and Stories*, ed. Cherisse W. Miller (Rockville, MD: Association of Adult Musicians with Hearing Loss Publications, 2011), 4.

3. Andrew J. Oxenham, "The Perception of Musical Tones," in *The Psychology of Music*, 3rd ed., ed. Diana Deutsch (Amsterdam: Academic Press, 2013), 18.

4. See Nina Kraus and Trent Nicol, "The Musician's Auditory World," *Acoustics Today* 6/3 (July 2010): 15–26, for an overview of recent findings concerning this connection. See also Nina Kraus, "Playing Music to Improve Hearing in Noise and Tune the Brain," *ENT and Audiology News* 22/3 (July/August 2013): 92–93.

5. Albert S. Bregman, *Auditory Scene Analysis: The Perceptual Organization of Sound* (Cambridge, MA: MIT Press, 1990), 5–6.

6. Ibid., 6.

7. See ibid., 38–43, for a discussion of innate versus learned segregation of *auditory streams*: the term Bregman uses to describe meaningfully distinct packages of auditory information.

8. Ibid., 457.

9. Ibid., 17–18.

10. Ibid., 643.

11. Ibid., 17–18.

12. Jay Alan Zimmerman, "Beethoven and Me: The Effects of Hearing-Loss on Music Composition," *Canadian Hearing Report* 8/2 (2013): 37.

13. Bregman, *Auditory Scene Analysis*, 461–64.

14. In "'How to Truly Listen'? Resisting an Idealized Sense of the Deaf Body," a paper presented at the American Musicological Society's annual meeting in Louisville, Kentucky, in 2015, Jessica Holmes warned against sensationalizing the evidence for neuroplasticity in the adult brain. In her recent article "Expert Listening Beyond the Limits of Hearing: Music and Deafness," *Journal of the American Musicological Society* 70 (2017): 171-220, Holmes argues for a broad and diversified understanding of listening experiences among the deaf, using the idealized cultural perception of percussionist Evelyn Glennie as a starting point for developing a more nuanced set of views based on the experiences of a wide range of subjects. While the information I present in the remainder of this chapter is anecdotal and may be limited to a small subset of people with hearing loss, I believe it is nevertheless relevant to understanding Beethoven, who, like Barbara, was postlingually deaf and who, like the others cited here, had extensive musical training before his hearing loss.

15. Post to ClarionCI@yahoogroups.com, February 3, 2005.

16. Kate Gfeller, "Music Perception of Cochlear Implant Recipients and Implications for Counseling and (Re)habilitation," *Perspectives on Hearing and Hearing Disorders: Research and Diagnostics* 16 (December 2012): 64. In a fascinating article, "Do Signals Have Politics? Inscribing Abilities in Cochlear Implants," in *The Oxford Handbook of Sound Studies*, ed. T. J. Pinch and Karen Bijsterveld (New York: Oxford University Press, 2012), 320–46, Mara Mills shows how the preferences of early cochlear implant users came to determine the nature of the programming codes that were created for their use, which in turn became embedded in later codes, while the recommendations of later users were often ignored.

17. Huw R. Cooper and Brian Roberts, "Auditory Stream Segregation of Tone Sequences in Cochlear Implant Listeners," *Hearing Research* 225 (2007): 14.

18. Ibid., 23.

19. Arlene Romoff, *Hear Again: Back to Life with a Cochlear Implant* (New York: League for the Hard of Hearing Publications, 1999), 92.

20. Cherisse W. Miller, ed., *Making Music with a Hearing Loss: Strategies and Stories,* (Rockville, MD: Association of Adult Musicians with Hearing Loss Publications, 2011), 44.

21. Post to ClarionCI@yahoogroups.com, June 6, 2004.

22. Post to ClarionCI@yahoogroups.com, November 28, 2004.

23. Personal communication, November 3, 2015.

24. Ibid.

25. This observation about singing is based on a comment by Kristin Oberle posted January 16, 2016, on the Association of Adult Musicians with Hearing Loss blog, http://www.bigtent.com/group/forum/message/95780938?ff=1. Used by permission. In "Two Voices: Singers in the Hearing/Deaf Borderlands," a paper presented at the American Musicological Society's annual meeting in Louisville, KY, in 2015, Katherine Meizel discussed the widely varying ways that prominent deaf singers negotiate the challenge of performing with hearing loss. Meizel emphasized the diversity of their experiences, which has led T. L. Forsberg to argue for a "DeaF" identity, in which the capital *F* represents fluidity.

26. Thayer-Forbes, 565–66.

27. "Ueber Beethoven's Taubheit," *Niederrheinische Musik-Zeitung für Kunstfreunde und Künstler* 2 (1854): 213–14. My translation.

28. Miller, *Making Music with a Hearing Loss*, 24.

29. Ibid., 39.

30. Lewis Lockwood, *Beethoven: The Music and the Life* (New York: W. W. Norton, 2003), 389.

CHAPTER SEVEN

1. Joseph N. Straus, *Extraordinary Measures: Disability in Music* (Oxford: Oxford University Press, 2011), 21.

2. Joseph Kerman, ed., *Ludwig van Beethoven. Autograph Miscellany from circa 1786 to 1799: British Museum Additional Manuscript no. 29801, ff. 39–162 (The Kafka Sketchbook)* (London: British Museum, 1970), 1:xxvii.

3. Ibid., 1:xxxiii.

4. Ibid., 2:121–22. Kerman's transcriptions are the basis for examples 7.1a and b.

5. "Nachrichten. Wien.," *Allgemeine musikalische Zeitung* 28 (May 10, 1826): 310–11. My translation.

6. Senner, Wallace, and Meredith, *Critical Reception*, 1:142 (no. 63).

7. David B. Levy, "'Ma però beschleunigend': Notation and Meaning in Ops. 133/134," *Beethoven Forum* 14/2 (Fall 2007): 143–44. Levy also points out the puzzlement caused from the first by Beethoven's choice to notate the subject as a series of tied eighth notes when single quarter notes would have been sufficient—a notational choice he preserved in the piano transcription pub-

lished as Opus 134, and which Levy also traces to baroque rhetorical gestures associated with suffering.

8. Beethoven's painstaking arrival at this unique countersubject, as shown in the surviving sketches for the *Grosse Fuge*, is discussed in detail in William E. Caplin, "The Genesis of the Countersubjects for the *Grosse Fuge*," in *The String Quartets of Beethoven*, ed. William Kinderman (Urbana: University of Illinois Press, 2006), 234–61.

9. Igor Stravinsky and Robert Craft, *Dialogues and a Diary* (Garden City, NY: Doubleday, 1963), 24.

10. Senner, Wallace, and Meredith, *Critical Reception*, 2:52–53.

11. Leonard Ratner has also noted the heightened importance of texture in Opus 59, pointing out that "the aural effects of texture in the string quartet were complemented by visual impressions: the four players on a stage or in the center of a salon could easily be pictured as an opera buffa ensemble as they engaged in their play of sound and figure." Leonard G. Ratner, "Texture, A Rhetorical Element in Beethoven's Quartets," in *Israel Studies in Musicology* (Jerusalem: Israel Musicological Society, 1980), 2:52.

12. For an overview of the changes to the sonic environment of Europe caused by the Industrial Revolution, see R. Murray Schafer, *The Soundscape: Our Sonic Environment and the Tuning of the World* (Rochester, VT: Destiny Books, 1994), 71–87. On specific aspects of the transformation, see Olivier Balaÿ, "The 19th Century Transformation of the Urban Soundscape," in *Internoise 2007: The 36th International Congress and Exhibition on Noise Control Engineering; Global Approaches to Noise Control, Istanbul, September 2007,* CR-Rom (Istanbul: Internoise, 2007), 1–10; and Nicholas Mathew, "Urban Space, Spectacle, Memory and Music in Nineteenth-Century Vienna," http://globalurbanhumanities.berkeley.edu/urban-space-spectacle-memory-and-music-in-nineteenth-century-vienna, accessed March 1, 2016.

13. "News: From the Lower Rhine," in *The Critical Reception of Beethoven's Compositions by His German Contemporaries, op. 125*, ed. and trans. Robin Wallace (Boston: Center for Beethoven Research, Boston University, 2017), 26, http://www.bu.edu/beethovencenter/files/2017/06/robinwallace-publication.pdf.

14. "The Lower Rhine Music Festival, 1825 in Aachen," in ibid., 28.

15. Wallace, *Beethoven's Critics*, 48.

16. Adolf Bernhard Marx, "Recension: L. v. Beethoven Ouvertüre et Entr'actes de la Tragédie Egmont, arr. p. 2 Vlons, Alto et Vcelle—3 Fl. 30 Kr. Pour Piano et Violon par Alex. Brand 3 Fl. 12 Kr. Bei Schott in Mainz, Antwerpen und Paris," *Berliner allgemeine musikalische Zeitung* 4 (June 20, 1827): 194.

17. Senner, Wallace, and Meredith, *Critical Reception*, 2:96.

18. Ibid., 2:97.

19. Deirdre Loughridge, *Haydn's Sunrise, Beethoven's Shadow: Audiovisual Culture and the Emergence of Musical Romanticism* (Chicago: University of Chicago Press, 2016), 6–9.

20. Re this translation of *Geisterseher*, which I and others have previously translated as "visionaries," see ibid., 202–8.

21. Another interesting recent take on visual imagery in Beethoven is presented by Christopher Reynolds in *Wagner, Schumann, and the Lessons of Beethoven's Ninth* (Oakland: University of California Press, 2015). Reynolds points out that "the German word *Gegenbewegung*, which describes counterpoint in contrary motion, was also used to describe a common military maneuver, 'the strategic movement of columns and lines of troops against the enemy, according to the way war began to be practiced during the eighteenth century from Frederick the Great onward'" (9). Beethoven, he says, would have needed "little more than an adolescent boy's knowledge of toy soldier formations" to understand the nature of this maneuver and represent it in a battle piece like *Wellington's Victory* with contrapuntal lines moving in opposite directions (10). Reynolds suggests that when Beethoven used this practice extensively in the Ninth Symphony, particularly its first movement, later commentators like Wagner understood the visual metaphor and drew on it to describe the music as a struggle between a protagonist striving for joy and a malevolent opponent who offers ongoing resistance (6). What Reynolds describes is more like traditional musical scene painting than the example from Loughridge, but he also believes that Beethoven developed a unique approach to conveying imagery through musical processes that deeply influenced later composers. See also his "The Representational Impulse in Late Beethoven, I: *An die ferne Geliebte*," *Acta Musicologica* 60 (1988): 43–61, and "The Representational Impulse in Late Beethoven, II: String Quartet in F Major, Op. 135," *Acta Musicologica* 60 (1988): 180–94.

22. Senner, Wallace, and Meredith, *Critical Reception*, 2:103.

23. See Senner, Wallace, and Meredith, *Critical Reception*, vol. 2, no. 149 (*Eroica*) and 219 (*Pastoral*). See also "Recension: *Siebente grosse Symphonie, in A dur, von Ludwig van Beethoven. 92stes Werk. Vollständige Partitur. Eigenthum der Verleger.* Wien bey S. A. Steiner u. Comp," *Allgemeine musikalische Zeitung* 18 (1816): 817–22, and "Recension: *Siebente grosse Symphonie, in A dur, von Ludwig van Beethoven. (92stes Werk.) Vollständige Partitur; dem Hochgebornen Herrn Moritz Reichsgrafen von Fries zugeeignet. (Eigenthum der Ver-*

leger.) Wien bey S. A. Steiner und Comp," *Allgemeine musikalische Zeitung mit besonderer Rücksicht auf den österreichischen Kaiserstaat* 1 (1817): 25–27, 37–40 (Seventh Symphony); "Recension: *Achte grosse Symphonie in F dur für 2 Violinen, 2 Violen, 2 Flauten, 2 Oboen, 2 Klarinetten, 2 Fagotte, 2 Hörner, 2 Trompeten, Pauken, Violoncell und Bass, von Ludwig van Beethoven.* 93stes Werk. Wien, bey Steiner und Comp," *Allgemeine musikalische Zeitung* 20 (1818): 161–67, and "Recension: *Achte grosse Sinfonie, (in F-dur).* Für 2 Violinen, 2 Violen, 2 Flöten, 2 Hoboen, 2 Trompeten, Pauken, Violoncell und Bass, von *Ludwig van Beethoven.* (93stes Werk.) Wien, im Verlage bey S. A. Steiner und Comp," *Allgemeine musikalische Zeitung mit besonderer Rücksicht auf den österreichischen Kaiserstaat* 2 (1818): 17–23 (Eighth Symphony).

24. Joseph Fröhlich, "First Review," in *Critical Reception of Beethoven's Compositions by His German Contemporaries, op. 125,* ed. Wallace, 59.

25. Friedrich Rochlitz, "Auf Veranlassung von: 1. Grand Quatour—pour deux Violons, Alto et Violoncelle, comp.——par Louis van Beethoven. Oeuvr. 131. Mayence, chez les fils de B. Schott. (Preis 4 Fl. 30 Xr.) 2. Grand Quatour—en partition—(Pr. 2 Fl. 42 Xr.)," *Allgemeine musikalische Zeitung* 30 (July 23 and 30, 1828), 485–95 and 501–9. My translation.

26. Quoted and translated in Sir George Grove, *Beethoven and His Nine Symphonies* (London: Novello, 1903), 244.

27. Carl Friedrich Ebers, "Reflexionen," *Caecilia* 2 (1825): 271. My translation.

28. Ibid., 272. My translation.

EPILOGUE

1. Thayer-Forbes, 777.

2. Thayer-Forbes, 115.

3. Parker Palmer, *Let Your Life Speak: Listening for the Voice of Vocation* (San Francisco: Jossey-Bass, 2000), 66.

4. These remarks appear in Palmer's unedited interview with Krista Tippett for the February 26, 2009, episode of *On Being,* https://onbeing.org/programs/parker-palmer-andrew-solomon-and-anita-barrows-the-soul-in-depression/.

5. Senner, Wallace, and Meredith, *Critical Reception,* 2:97. Elsewhere I have written about this aspect of Beethoven's music in considerable detail; see Robin Wallace, "Background and Expression in the First Movement of Beethoven's Op. 132," *Journal of Musicology* 7 (Winter 1989): 3–20, and "Myth, Gender, and Musical Meaning: *The Magic Flute,* Beethoven, and 19th-Century Sonata Form Revisited," *Journal of Musicological Research* 19 (1999): 1–25.

6. Scott Burnham, *Beethoven Hero* (Princeton, NJ: Princeton University Press, 1995), 167.

7. In my essay "The Deaf Composer and His Broadwood: A Working Relationship," in *Inside the Hearing Machine*, 46, I apply this same idea to the first parts of both halves of the fourth (double) variation in the last movement of Opus 111, Beethoven's last piano sonata.

Bibliography

Albrecht, Theodore, trans. and ed. *Beethoven's Conversation Books*. 12 vols. Martlesham, Suffolk, UK: Boydell and Brewer, forthcoming beginning fall 2018.

———. "The Fortnight Fallacy: A Revised Chronology for Beethoven's *Christ on the Mount of Olives*, Op. 85, and Wielhorsky Sketchbook." *Journal of Musicological Research* 11 (1991): 1–22.

Asherson, Nehemiah. "The Deafness of Beethoven and the Saga of the Stapes." *Transactions of the Hunterian Society* 24 (1965–66): 7–34.

Balaÿ, Olivier. "The 19th Century Transformation of the Urban Soundscape." In *Internoise 2007: The 36th International Congress and Exhibition on Noise Control Engineering. Global Approaches to Noise Control, Istanbul, September 2007*, CR-Rom, 1–10. Istanbul: Internoise, 2007.

Bankl, Hans, and Hans Jesserer. *Die Krankheiten Ludwig van Beethovens*. Vienna: Wilhelm Maudrich, 1987.

Beethoven, Ludwig van. *Beethoven: String Quartet Opus 59 No. 1 (First "Razumovsky" Quartet, in F major)*. Edited by Alan Tyson. London: Scolar, 1980.

Beghin, Tom. "Beethoven's *Hammerklavier* Sonata, Opus 106: Legend, Difficulty, and the Gift of a Broadwood Piano." *Keyboard Perspectives* 7 (2014): 81–121.

———. "Three Builders, Two Pianos, One Pianist: The Told and Untold Story of Ignaz Moscheles's Concert on 15 December 1823." *19th-Century Music* 24/2 (Autumn 2000): 115–48.

———. *The Virtual Haydn: Paradox of a Twenty-First-Century Keyboardist*. Chicago: University of Chicago Press, 2015.

Bennion, Elisabeth. *Antique Hearing Devices*. London: Vernier, 1994.

Blondel, Raoul. "La surdité de Beethoven." *Le Ménestrel* 90 (1928): 173–74.

Blume, Stuart. *The Artificial Ear: Cochlear Implants and the Culture of Deafness*. New Brunswick, NJ: Rutgers University Press, 2010.

Böhme, G. "Wie wurde Ludwig van Beethovens Hörstörung behandelt?" *Audio-Symposium / Bommer International Rexton Hearing Aids* 4 (1977): 25–38.

Brandenburg, Sieghard, ed. *Ludwig van Beethoven: Briefwechsel Gesamtausgabe*. 7 vols. Munich: G. Henle, 1996.

Bregman, Albert S. *Auditory Scene Analysis: The Perceptual Organization of Sound*. Cambridge: MIT Press, 1990.

———. "Progress in Understanding Auditory Scene Analysis." *Music Perception* 33/1 (September 2015): 12–19.

Breuning, Gerhard von. *Aus dem Schwarzspanierhause: Erinnerungen an L. van Beethoven aus seiner Jugendzeit*. Neudruck mit Ergänzungen und Erläuterungen von Dr. Alfr. Chr. Kalischer. Berlin: Schuster und Loeffler, 1907.

Burnham, Scott. *Beethoven Hero*. Princeton, NJ: Princeton University Press, 1995.

Caplin, William E. "The Genesis of the Countersubjects for the *Grosse Fuge*." In *The String Quartets of Beethoven*, ed. William Kinderman, 234–61. Urbana: University of Illinois Press, 2006.

Chasin, Marshall, ed. *Hearing Loss in Musicians: Prevention and Management*. San Diego: Plural, 2009.

Chorost, Michael. "My Bionic Quest for Boléro." *Wired*, November 1, 2005, http://www.wired.com/2005/11/bolero/, accessed October 26, 2017.

———. *Rebuilt: My Journey Back to the Hearing World*. Boston: Houghton-Mifflin, 2005.

Cook, Nicholas. *Music: A Very Short Introduction*. Oxford: Oxford University Press, 1998.

Cooper, Barry, ed. *The Beethoven Compendium: A Guide to Beethoven's Life and Music*. London: Thames and Hudson, 1991.

———. "Beethoven's Oratorio and the Heiligenstadt Testament." *Beethoven Journal* 10/1 (Spring 1995): 19–24.

Cooper, Huw R., and Brian Roberts. "Auditory Stream Segregation of Tone Sequences in Cochlear Implant Listeners." *Hearing Research* 225 (2007): 11–24.

Cureoglu, Sebahattin, Muzeyyen Yildirim Baylan, and Michael M. Paparella. "Cochlear Otosclerosis." *Current Opinion in Otolaryngology & Head and Neck Surgery* 18/5 (Oct. 2010): 357–62.

Davies, Peter J. *Beethoven in Person: His Deafness, Illnesses, and Death.* Westport, CT: Greenwood, 2001.

———. "The Cause of Beethoven's Deafness." In *Aflame with Music: 100 Years of Music at the University of Melbourne,* edited by Brenton Broadstock et al., 143–51. Parkville, Victoria: Centre for Studies in Australian Music, 1996.

DeNora, Tia. *Beethoven and the Construction of Genius: Musical Politics in Vienna, 1792–1803.* Berkeley: University of California Press, 1995.

Dorfmüller, Kurt, Norbert Gertsch, and Julia Ronge, eds. *Ludwig van Beethoven: Thematisch-bibliographisches Werkverzeichnis.* Munich: G. Henle, 2014.

Dotter, Franz, and Ingeborg Okorn. "Austria's Hidden Conflict: Hearing Culture versus Deaf Culture." In *Many Ways to Be Deaf: International Variation in Deaf Communities,* edited by Leila Frances Monaghan et al., 49–66. Washington, DC: Gallaudet University Press, 2003.

Ealy, George Thomas. "Of Ear Trumpets and a Resonance Plate: Early Hearing Aids and Beethoven's Hearing Perception." *19th-Century Music* 17/3 (Spring 1994): 262–73.

Ebers, Carl Friedrich. "Reflexionen." *Caecilia* 2 (1825): 271–72.

"Einige Worte zu den vielen über Beethovens letzte Werke." *Allgemeine musikalische Zeitung* 31 (29 April 1829): 269–73.

Eisinger, Josef. "Was Beethoven Lead-Poisoned?" *Beethoven Journal* 23/1 (Summer 2008): 15–17.

F. "*Das Neiderrheinische Musikfest,* 1825 in Aachen." *Caecilia* 4 (1826): 63–70.

Frimmel, Theodor von. "Beethovens Taubheit." In *Beethoven-Forschung: Lose Blätter,* edited by Theodor von Frimmel, 1:82–99. Vienna: Kommissions-Verlag Gerold, 1912.

Fröhlich, Joseph, and Georg Christian Grossheim. "Sinfonie, mit Schlusschor über Schillers Ode: 'An die Freude,' für grosses Orchester, 4 Solo- und 4 Chor-Stimmen, componirt von *Ludwig van Beethoven.* 125tes Werk. . . . Zwei Recensionen." *Caecilia* 9 (1828): 231–61.

Gfeller, Kate. "Music Perception of Cochlear Implant Recipients and Implications for Counseling and (Re)habilitation." *Perspectives on Hearing and Hearing Disorders: Research and Diagnostics* 16 (December 2012): 64–73.

Gfeller, Kate, et al. "Musical Backgrounds, Listening Habits, and Aesthetic Enjoyment of Adult Cochlear Implant Recipients." *Journal of the American Academy of Audiology* 11 (2000): 390–406.

Gjerdingen, Robert O. *Music in the Galant Style.* Oxford: Oxford University Press, 2007.

Good, Edwin M. *Giraffes, Black Dragons, and Other Pianos: A Technological History from Cristofori to the Modern Concert Grand*. 2nd ed. Stanford, CA: Stanford University Press, 2001.

Grossheim, Christian Georg, and Joseph Fröhlich. "Missa composita a Ludovico v. Beethoven, Op. 123. . . . Zwei Recensionen." *Caecilia* 9 (1828): 22–45.

Grove, Sir George. *Beethoven and His Nine Symphonies*. London: Novello, 1903.

Hain, Timothy C. "Otosclerosis." http://www.dizziness-and balance.com /disorders/hearing/otoscler.html, accessed February 18, 2015.

Herre, Grita, ed. *Beethoven im Gespräch: Ein Konversationsheft vom 9. September 1825*. Bonn: Verlag Beethoven-Haus, 2002.

Holmes, Jessica. "Expert Listening beyond the Limits of Hearing: Music and Deafness." *Journal of the American Musicological Society* 70 (2017): 171–220.

———."'How to Truly Listen'? Resisting an Idealized Sense of the Deaf Body." Paper delivered at the annual meeting of the American Musicological Society, Louisville, KY, 2015.

Hong, Robert S., and Christopher W. Turner. "Pure-Tone Auditory Stream Segregation and Speech Perception in Noise in Cochlear Implant Recipients." *Journal of the Acoustical Society of America* 120/1 (July 2006): 360–74.

Hui, A. C. F., and S. M. Wong. "Deafness and Liver Disease in a 57-Year-Old Man: A Medical History of Beethoven." *Hong Kong Medical Journal* 6/4 (December 2000): 433–38.

Huxtable, Ryan J. "The Deafness of Beethoven: A Paradigm of Hearing Problems." *Proceedings of the Western Pharmacology Society* 43 (2000): 1–8.

Hyperacusis Network. "Decreased Sound Tolerance." http://www .hyperacusis.net/what-to-do/, accessed July 26, 2017.

Inside the Hearing Machine: Beethoven on His Broadwood; Piano Sonatas Opus 109, 110, and 111. N.p.: Evil Penguin Records Classic, 2017.

Jander, Owen. "The Rhetorical Structure of Beethoven's Heiligenstadt Testament." *Beethoven Journal* 22/1 (Summer 2007): 6–16.

Jerold, Beverly. "Mälzel's Role in Beethoven's Symphonic Metronome Marks." In *Music Performance Issues: 1600–1900*, 165–92. Hillsdale, NY: Pendragon, 2016.

Johnson, Douglas, Alan Tyson, and Robert Winter. *The Beethoven Sketchbooks: History, Reconstruction, Inventory*. Berkeley: University of California Press, 1985.

Kanne, Friedrich August. "Academie des Lud. van Beethoven." *Allgemeine musikalische Zeitung mit besonderen Rücksicht auf den österreichischen Kaiserstaat* 8 (June 5, 9, and 16, 1824): 149–51, 157–60, 173–74.

Karmody, Collin S., and Edgar S. Bachor. "The Deafness of Ludwig van Beethoven: An Immunopathy." *Otology and Neurotology* 26/4 (July 2005): 809–14.

Kerman, Joseph. "Beethoven's Early Sketches." *Musical Quarterly* 56 (1970): 515–38.

———, ed. *Ludwig van Beethoven. Autograph Miscellany from circa 1786 to 1799: British Museum Additional Manuscript no. 29801, ff. 39–162 (The Kafka Sketchbook)*. London: British Museum, 1970.

Kinderman, William, ed. *Artaria 195: Beethoven's Sketchbook for the "Missa Solemnis" and the Piano Sonata in E Major, Opus 109*. 3 vols. Urbana: University of Illinois Press, 2003.

———. *Beethoven*. Berkeley: University of California Press, 1995.

———, ed. *Beethoven's Compositional Process*. Lincoln: University of Nebraska Press, 1991.

Klinger, Wolfram. "Das Rätsel von Beethovens Gehörleiden." *Bonner Beethoven-Studien* 5 (2006): 119–41.

Knittel, K. M. "Pilgrimages to Beethoven: Reminiscences by His Contemporaries." *Music and Letters* 84 (2003): 19–54.

———. "Wagner, Deafness, and the Reception of Beethoven's Late Style." *Journal of the American Musicological Society* 51 (1998): 49–82.

Koelkebeck, Mary Lou, Colleen Detjen, and Donald R. Calvert. *Historic Devices for Hearing: The CID-Goldstein Collection*. Saint Louis, MO: Central Institute for the Deaf, 1984.

Köhler, Karl-Heinz and Grita Herre, eds. *Ludwig van Beethovens Konversationshefte*. 11 vols. Leipzig: Deutscher Verlag für Musik, 1972–2001.

Kopitz, Klaus Martin, and Rainer Cadenbach, eds. *Beethoven aus der Sicht seiner Zeitgenossen in Tagebüchern, Briefen, Gedichten und Erinnerungen*. 2 vols. Munich: G. Henle, 2009.

Kraus, Beate Angelika. *Beethoven-Rezeption in Frankreich: Von ihren Anfängen bis zum Untergang des Second Empire*. Bonn: Verlag Beethoven-Haus, 2001.

Kraus, Nina. "Playing Music to Improve Hearing in Noise and Tune the Brain." *ENT and Audiology News* 22/3 (July/August 2013): 92–93.

Kraus, Nina, and Samira Anderson. "Hearing with Our Brains." *Hearing Journal* 65/9 (September 2012): 48.

Kraus, Nina, and Trent Nicol. "The Musician's Auditory World." *Acoustics Today* 6/3 (July 2010): 15–26.

Landon, H. C. Robbins. *Beethoven: A Documentary Study*. London: Thames and Hudson, 1970.

Larkin, Edward. "Beethoven's Medical History." In Martin Cooper, *Beetho-*

ven: *The Last Decade: 1817–1827*, 439–66. London: Oxford University Press, 1970.

Levy, David B. "'Ma però beschleunigend': Notation and Meaning in Ops. 133/134." *Beethoven Forum* 14/2 (Fall 2007): 129–49.

Lockwood, Lewis. *Beethoven: Studies in the Creative Process*. Cambridge, MA: Harvard University Press, 1992.

———. *Beethoven: The Music and the Life*. New York: W. W. Norton, 2003.

———. "The Three Years 1813–1817: A 'Fallow' Period in Beethoven's Career?" In *Beiträge zu Biographie und Schaffensprozess bei Beethoven, Rainer Cadenbach zum Gedenken*, edited by Jürgen May, 89–99. Bonn: Verlag Beethoven-Haus, 2011.

Lockwood, Lewis, and Alan Gosman, eds. *Beethoven's "Eroica" Sketchbook: A Critical Edition*. 2 vols. Urbana: University of Illinois Press, 2013.

Looi, Valerie, Kate Gfeller, and Virginia D. Driscoll. "Music Appreciation and Training for Cochlear Implant Recipients: A Review." *Seminars in Hearing* 33 (2012): 307–44.

Loughridge, Dierdre. *Haydn's Sunrise, Beethoven's Shadow: Audiovisual Culture and the Emergence of Musical Romanticism*. Chicago: University of Chicago Press, 2016.

Marage [no first name given]. "Causes et conséquences de la surdité de Beethoven." Transmitted by d'Arsonvale. *Comptes Rendus des Séances Hebdomadaires de l'Académie des Sciences* 189 (1929): 1036–38.

Marston, Nicholas. *Beethoven's Piano Sonata in E, Op. 109*. Oxford: Clarendon, 1995.

Marx, Adolph Bernhard. "Recension. L. v. Beethoven Ouvertüre et Entr'actes de la Tragédie Egmont, arr. p. 2 Vlons, Alto et Vcelle—3 Fl. 30 Kr. Pour Piano et Violon par Alex. Brand 3 Fl. 12 Kr. Bei Schott in Mainz, Antwerpen und Paris." *Berliner allgemeine musikalische Zeitung* 4 (20 June 1827): 194.

———. *Ueber Malerei in der Tonkunst: Ein Maigruß an die Kunstphilosophen*. Berlin: G. Finck, 1828.

Mathew, Nicholas. "Urban Space, Spectacle, Memory and Music in Nineteenth-Century Vienna." http://globalurbanhumanities.berkeley.edu/urban-space-spectacle-memory-and-music-in-nineteenth-century-vienna, accessed March 1, 2016.

McCabe, Brian F. "Beethoven's Deafness." *Annals of Otology, Rhinology and Laryngology* 67/1 (March 1958): 192–206.

Meizel, Katherine. "Two Voices: Singers in the Hearing/Deaf Borderlands." Paper delivered at the annual meeting of the American Musicological Society, Louisville, KY, 2015.

Miller, Alice. *The Drama of the Gifted Child*. Translated from the German by Ruth Ward. New York: Basic Books, 1990.

Miller, Cherisse W., ed. *Making Music with a Hearing Loss: Strategies and Stories*. Rockville, MD: Association of Adult Musicians with Hearing Loss Publications, 2011.

Mills, Mara. "Do Signals Have Politics? Inscribing Abilities in Cochlear Implants." In *The Oxford Handbook of Sound Studies,* edited by T. J. Pinch and Karen Bijsterveld, 320–46. New York: Oxford University Press, 2012.

———. "Hearing Aids and the History of Electronics Miniaturization." *IEEE Annals of the History of Computing* (April-June 2011): 25–44.

———. "When Mobile Communication Technologies Were New." *Endeavour* 33/4 (2009): 140–46.

Mobbs, Kenneth. "A Performer's Comparative Study of Touchweight, Key-Dip, Keyboard Design and Repetition in Early Grand Pianos, c. 1770 to 1850." *Galpin Society Journal* 54 (May 2001): 16–54.

Mom, Thierry, et al. "Cochlear Blood Supply: An Update on Anatomy and Function." *Fr ORL* 2005: 81–88. http://citeseerx.ist.psu.edu/viewdoc/download?doi=10.1.1.472.3787&rep=rep1&type=pdf, accessed October 21, 2017.

Mudry, Albert, and Mara Mills. "The Early History of the Cochlear Implant: A Retrospective." *JAMA Otolaryngology—Head Neck Surgery* 139/5 (May 2013): 446–53.

"Nachrichten. *Vom Niederrhein*." *Allgemeine musikalische Zeitung* 25 (1825): 444–49.

"Nachrichten: *Wien*." *Allgemeine musikalische Zeitung* 28 (May 10, 1826): 310–11.

Newman, William S. *Beethoven on Beethoven: Playing His Piano Music His Way*. New York: W. W. Norton, 1988.

Oxenham, Andrew J. "The Perception of Musical Tones." In *The Psychology of Music*, 3rd ed., edited by Diana Deutsch, 1–33. Amsterdam: Academic Press, 2013.

Palmer, Parker. *Let Your Life Speak: Listening for the Voice of Vocation*. San Francisco: Jossey-Bass, 2000.

Palmer, Parker, Andrew Solomon, and Anita Barrows. "The Soul in Depression." *On Being*, May 1, 2003. https://onbeing.org/programs/parker-palmer-andrew-solomon-and-anita-barrows-the-soul-in-depression/.

Politzer, Adam. *A Text-Book of the Diseases of the Ear and Adjacent Organs*. Translated and edited by James Patterson Cassells. Philadelphia: Henry C. Lea's Son, 1883.

Radiolab. "Colors." Season 10, episode 13. http://www.radiolab.org/story /211119-colors/.

Ratner, Leonard G. "Texture, a Rhetorical Element in Beethoven's Quartets." In *Israel Studies in Musicology*, 2:51–76. Jerusalem: Israel Musicological Society, 1980.

"Recension: *Achte grosse Sinfonie, (in F-dur).* Für 2 Violinen, 2 Violen, 2 Flöten, 2 Hoboen, 2 Trompeten, Pauken, Violoncell und Bass, von *Ludwig van Beethoven.* (93stes Werk.) Wien, im Verlage bey S. A. Steiner und Comp." *Allgemeine musikalische Zeitung mit besonderer Rücksicht auf den österreichischen Kaiserstaat* 2 (1818): 17–23.

"Recension: *Achte grosse Symphonie in F dur für 2 Violinen, 2 Violen, 2 Flauten, 2 Oboen, 2 Klarinetten, 2 Fagotte, 2 Hörner, 2 Trompeten, Pauken, Violoncell und Bass, von Ludwig van Beethoven.* 93stes Werk. Wien, bey Steiner und Comp." *Allgemeine musikalische Zeitung* 20 (1818): 161–67.

"Recension: *Phantasie für das Pianoforte, mit Begleitung des ganzen Orchesters und Chor, in Musik gesetzt——von Louis van Beethoven. 8ostes Werk.* (Eigenthum der Verleger.) Leipzig, bey Breitkopf und Härtel. (Preis 2 Thlr. 12 Gr.)." *Allgemeine musikalische Zeitung* 14 (May 6, 1812): 307–11.

"Recension: *Quatour pour 2 Violons, Viola et Violencelle comp.—par L. v. Beethoven.* Oeuv. 74. A Leipsic, chez Breitkopf et Härtel. (Preis 1 Thlr. 8 Gr.)." *Allgemeine musikalische Zeitung* 13 (May 22, 1811): 349–51.

"Recension: *Siebente grosse Symphonie, in A dur, von Ludwig van Beethoven.* (92stes Werk.) Vollständige Partitur; dem Hochgebornen Herrn Moritz Reichsgrafen von Fries zugeeignet. (Eigenthum der Verleger.) Wien bey S. A. Steiner und Comp." *Allgemeine musikalische Zeitung mit besonderer Rücksicht auf den österreichischen Kaiserstaat* 1 (1817): 25–27, 37–40.

"Recension: *Siebente grosse Symphonie, in A dur, von Ludwig van Beethoven.* 92stes Werk. Vollständige Partitur. Eigenthum der Verleger. Wien bey S. A. Steiner u. Comp." *Allgemeine musikalische Zeitung* 18 (1816): 817–22.

"Recensionen: *Wellington's Sieg, oder, die Schlacht bey Vittoria, in Musik gesetzt, und Sr. königl. Hoheit, dem Prinzen Regenten von England—zugeeignet, von Ludwig van Beethoven.* 91stes Werk. Vollständige Partitur. (Und die mannigfaltigen Ausgaben, wie sie in der Folge angeführt werden.) Wien, bey S. A. Steiner und Comp., so wie auch in den vorzüglichsten Musikhandlungen Deutschlands, der Schweiz, und Italiens." *Allgemeine musikalische Zeitung* 18 (April 10, 1816): 241–50.

"Rezensionen neuer Musikalien. Fantaisie pour le Pianoforte composée et dediée—par L. v. Beethoven Oeuv. 77 à Vienne chez Jean Cappi." *Wiener allgemeine musikalische Zeitung* 1 (March 27, 1813): 197–99.

Reynolds, Christopher. "The Representational Impulse in Late Beethoven, I: *An die ferne Geliebte*." *Acta Musicologica* 60 (1988): 43–61.

———. "The Representational Impulse in Late Beethoven, II: String Quartet in F Major, Op. 135." *Acta Musicologica* 60 (1988): 180–94.

———. *Wagner, Schumann, and the Lessons of Beethoven's Ninth*. Oakland: University of California Press, 2015.

Rochlitz, Friedrich. "Auf Veranlassung von: 1. Grand Quatour—pour deux Violons, Alto et Violoncelle, comp.—par Louis van Beethoven. Oeuvr. 131. Mayence, chez les fils de B. Schott. (Preis 4 Fl. 30 Xr.) 2. Grand Quatour—en partition—(Pr. 2 Fl. 42 Xr.)." *Allgemeine musikalische Zeitung* 30 (July 23 and 30, 1828): 485–95, 501–9.

———. "Schreiben Mozarts an den Baron von . . ." *Allgemeine musikalische Zeitung* 17 (August 23, 1815): col. 563–64.

Rolland, Romain. *Beethoven the Creator*. Translated by Ernest Newman. New York: Harper and Brothers, 1929.

Romoff, Arlene. *Hear Again: Back to Life with a Cochlear Implant*. New York: League for the Hard of Hearing Publications, 1999.

———. *Listening Closely: A Journey to Bilateral Hearing*. Watertown, MA: Imagine! Publishing, 2011.

Rose, Maria. "New Insights into Beethoven's 'Waldstein' Sonata Op. 53: A Showpiece for Paris." Paper delivered at the annual meeting of the American Musicological Society, Pittsburgh, 2013.

Ross, Megan. "Beethoven's Late Quartets and Wagner's 1870 'Beethoven' Essay Revisited." Paper delivered at the Seventh New Beethoven Research Conference, Rochester, NY, 2017.

Sacks, Oliver. *Migraine: Understanding a Common Disorder*. Expanded and updated ed. Berkeley: University of California Press, 1985.

Schafer, Hollace Ann. "'A Wisely Ordered *Phantasie*': Joseph Haydn's Creative Process from the Sketches and Drafts for Instrumental Music." Ph.D. diss., Brandeis University, 1987.

Schafer, R. Murray. *The Soundscape: Our Sonic Environment and the Tuning of the World*. Rochester, VT: Destiny Books, 1994.

Schindler, Anton F. *Biographie von Ludwig van Beethoven*. Münster: Aschendorff, 1840.

———. "Zur Beantwortung der Fragen über Beethoven's Taubheit, in Nr. 54 dieses Blattes." *Niederrheinische Musik-Zeitung für Kunstfreunde und Künstler* 2 (1854): 223–24.

Schweisheimer, Waldemar. *Beethovens Leiden: Ihr Einfluss auf sein Leben und Schaffen*. Munich: Georg Müller, 1922.

Scorsby, Maurice. "Beethoven's Deafness." *Journal of Laryngology and Otology* 45 (1930): 529–44.

Senner, Wayne, Robin Wallace, and William Meredith, eds. *The Critical Reception of Beethoven's Compositions by his German Contemporaries.* 2 vols. Lincoln: University of Nebraska Press, 1999, 2001.

Seyfried, Ignaz Xaver. "Recension[en]: I. L. van Beethoven: Messe solennelle, en *ré* majeur; Oeuv. 123. II. L. van Beethoven: Sinfonie, en *ré* mineur; Oeuv. 125. III. L. van Beethoven: Grand Quatour, en *ut-dièze* mineur, (*cis*-moll) pour deux Violons, Alto et Violoncelle; Oeuv. 131." *Caecilia* 9 (1828): 217–43.

Skowroneck, Tilman. *Beethoven the Pianist.* Cambridge: Cambridge University Press, 2010.

———. "Beethoven's Erard Piano: Its Influence on His Compositions and on Viennese Fortepiano Building." *Early Music* 30 (2002): 522–38.

———. "A Brit in Vienna: Beethoven's Broadwood Piano." *Keyboard Perspectives* 5 (2012): 41–82.

———. "Keyboard Instruments of the Young Beethoven." In *Beethoven and His World*, edited by Scott Burnham and Michael P. Steinberg, 151–92. Princeton, NJ: Princeton University Press, 2000.

Solomon, Maynard. *Beethoven Essays.* Cambridge, MA: Harvard University Press, 1988.

———. "Beethoven's Tagebuch of 1812–1818." In *Beethoven Studies 3*, edited by Alan Tyson, 193–285. Cambridge: Cambridge University Press, 1982.

———. "On Beethoven's Creative Process: A Two-Part Invention." *Music and Letters* 61 (1980): 272–83.

Sonneck, O. G., ed. *Beethoven: Impressions by His Contemporaries.* New York: Dover, 1967.

Squires, Paul C. "The Problem of Beethoven's Deafness." *Journal of Abnormal and Social Psychology* 32 (1937): 11–62.

Steblin, Rita. "Mälzel's Early Career to 1813: New Archival Research in Regensburg and Vienna." In *Colloquium Collegarum: Festschrift für David Hiley zum 65. Geburtstag*, edited by Wolfgang Horn and Fabian Weber, 161–210. Tutzing, Germany: Hans Schneider, 2013.

Stevens, Kenneth M., and William G. Hemingway. "Beethoven's Deafness." *Journal of the American Medical Association* 213/3 (July 20, 1970): 436–37.

Stevens, Michael H., Teemarie Jacobsen, and Alicia Kay Crofts. "Lead and the Deafness of Ludwig van Beethoven." *Laryngoscope* 123 (2013): 2855.

Straus, Joseph N. "Disability and 'Late Style' in Music." *Journal of Musicology* 25/1 (Winter 2008): 3–45.

———. *Extraordinary Measures: Disability in Music.* Oxford: Oxford University Press, 2011.

———. "Normalizing the Abnormal: Disability in Music and Music Theory." *Journal of the American Musicological Society* 59/1 (Spring 2006): 113–84.

Stravinsky, Igor. *Dialogues and a Diary.* Garden City, NY: Doubleday, 1963.

Thayer, Alexander Wheelock. *The Life of Ludwig van Beethoven.* Edited and revised by Henry Edward Krehbiel. 3 vols. New York: G. Schirmer, 1921.

Thayer, Alexander Wheelock. *Thayer's Life of Beethoven.* Revised and edited by Elliott Forbes. Princeton, NJ: Princeton University Press, 1967.

Tyson, Alan. "Beethoven's Heroic Phase." *Musical Times* 110 (February 1969): 139–41.

———. "Ferdinand Ries (1784–1838): The History of His Contribution to Beethoven Biography." *19th-Century Music* 7/3 (April 1984): 209–21.

"Ueber Beethoven's Taubheit." *Niederrheinische Musik-Zeitung für Kunstfreunde und Künstler* 2 (1854): 213–14.

Wallace, Robin. "Background and Expression in the First Movement of Beethoven's Op. 132." *Journal of Musicology* 7 (Winter 1989): 3–20.

———. *Beethoven's Critics: Aesthetic Dilemmas and Resolutions during the Composer's Lifetime.* Cambridge: Cambridge University Press, 1986.

———. "Myth, Gender, and Musical Meaning: *The Magic Flute*, Beethoven, and 19th-Century Sonata Form Revisited." *Journal of Musicological Research* 19 (1999): 1–25.

———, ed. and trans. *The Critical Reception of Beethoven's Compositions by His German Contemporaries, Op. 125.* Boston: Center for Beethoven Research, Boston University, 2017. http://www.bu.edu/beethovencenter/files/2017/06/robinwallace-publication.pdf.

Wawruch, Andreas Ignaz. "Medical Review on the Final Stage of L. van Beethoven's Life." Translated by Michael Lorenz. *Beethoven Journal* 22/2 (Winter 2007): 87–91.

Weber, Gottfried. "Ueber Tonmalerei." *Caecilia* 3, no. 10 (1825): 125–72.

Wegeler, Franz, and Ferdinand Ries. *Beethoven Remembered: The Biographical Notes of Franz Wegeler and Ferdinand Ries.* Arlington, VA: Great Ocean, 1987.

White-Schwoch, Travis, et al. "Older Adults Benefit from Music Training Early in Life: Biological Evidence for Long-Term Training-Driven Plasticity." *Journal of Neuroscience* 33/45 (November 6. 2013): 17667–74.

Woldemar, Ernst. "Aufforderung an die Redaktion der Cäcilia." *Caecilia* 8 (1828): 36–40.

Yule, Lawrence. "Cupped Hand Amplification." Solent Acoustics. https://
solentacoustics.wordpress.com/2014/06/17/cupped-hand-amplification/,
accessed March 29, 2017.

Zimmerman, Jay Alan. "Beethoven and Me: The Effects of Hearing-Loss on
Music Composition." *Canadian Hearing Report* 8/2 (2013): 35–39.

Index

Barbara's cochlear implants (*continued*)
music and, 98, 102, 104–5, 167–70,
171–72; remapping and, 97, 98–99;
settings for various situations and,
98–100; telephone conversations
and, 166–67. *See also* Barbara's hearing and communication tools; cochlear implants; Wallace, Barbara
Barbara's deafness and hearing loss:
Barbara's speaking volume and,
80; cause of, 39, 44, 47–48, 50, 54;
church and, 55, 170; denial of, 43,
44; family life and, 87–88, 105–6;
group conversations and, 81, 86–87,
106; house hunting and, 81; loss of
depth perception and, 164–65; loss
of hearing in left ear and, 3–4, 52–
54; loss of hearing in right ear and,
2–3, 47–48, 78, 86; mental Rolodex
and, 170; noisy environments and,
95–96; pitch of speaker's voice and,
44; progression of, 42–43; residual
hearing and, 82–83; simple vs. complex sounds and, 121; social isolation and, 4, 43, 55, 56, 87, 95–96, 213;
tactile vocal memory and, 84, 85;
television and, 80; tinnitus and, 43–
44, 91; treatment of, 39, 48, 50–51,
54; vacation experiences and, 211–
12. *See also* Barbara's cochlear implants; Barbara's hearing and communication tools; Wallace, Barbara
Barbara's hearing and communication
tools: ASL and, 56; in church, 83–
85; closed captioning and, 55; conversation books and writing things
down and, 3, 5, 55, 79–81, 85–86, 88,
95; cost of and insurance coverage
for, 44, 51, 90; FM system and, 52;

hearing aids and, 2, 42–43, 44–46;
instant messaging and, 55–56; lipreading and, 69, 70, 79, 83; pocket
talker and, 5, 8–9, 81–87, 82, 91, 95,
133, 165–66, 172. *See also* Barbara's
cochlear implants; Wallace, Barbara
Baylor Medical Center (Dallas, TX),
6, 90
Baylor University, 1, 2, 53, 81–82, 90
Beatles, 10
Beethoven, Caspar Carl van, 19, 29
Beethoven, Johanna van, 29
Beethoven, Karl van, 29–30, 141, 250–
51n79
Beethoven, Ludwig van: alcohol and,
17, 234n20; arrested as vagrant, 211–
12; childhood and education of,
28–29, 66, 223–24, 234n18; as conductor, 172–73, 207, 238n51; demys-
tification of, ix; depression and,
213–14, 215–16; fallow period of,
26–27, 237n48; heroic and tragic
stereotypes and, 217, 219–20; "heroic" middle period of, 26–27, 73,
113, 174–75, 219, 237n44; high expectations of, 213–14, 223–24; late
period of, 30–31, 71–75, 174–75;
legacy of, 175; love life of, 25–26, 27;
oeuvre of, 62, 223–24; as performer,
22, 26, 66–68, 117, 119, 240–41n9,
241nn10–11; vocation of, 77, 109;
wholeness and, 214, 216–17, 219–20,
222–24. *See also* Beethoven's composition process; Beethoven's deafness and hearing loss; Beethoven's
hearing and communication tools;
Beethoven's musical style; Beethoven's pianos; Beethoven's resonator; Beethoven's sketches and man-